Springer Japan KK

T. Nakano, S.Z. Goldhaber (Eds.)

Pulmonary Embolism

With 69 Figures

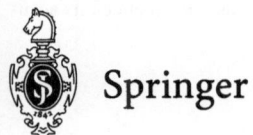 Springer

Takeshi Nakano, M.D.
Professor, The First Department of Internal Medicine
Mie University School of Medicine
174-2 Edobashi, Tsu, Mie 514-8507, Japan

Samuel Z. Goldhaber, M.D.
Associate Professor, Cardiovascular Division, Department of Medicine
Brigham and Woman's Hospital
Harvard Medical School
75 Francis Street, Boston, MA 02115, USA

ISBN 978-4-431-66895-4   ISBN 978-4-431-66893-0 (eBook)
DOI 10.1007/978-4-431-66893-0

Library of Congress Cataloging-in-Publication Data

Pulmonary embolism/T. Nakano, S.Z. Goldhaber (eds.).
    p. cm.
    Includes bibliographical references and index.
    ISBN 4-431-70238-5 (hard cover: alk. paper)
    1. Pulmonary embolism. I. Nakano, T. (Takeshi), 1942– . II. Goldhaber, Samuel Z.
    [DNLM: 1. Pulmonary Embolism. WG 420 P973 1999]
    RC776.P85P8232 1999
    616.2′49—dc21
    DNLM/DLC   99-24991
    for Library of Congress

Printed on acid-free paper

© Springer Japan 1999
Originally published by Springer-Verlag Tokyo in 1999
Softcover reprint of the hardcover 1st edition 1999
This work is subject to copyright. All rights are reserved, whether the whole or part of the material is concerned, specifically the rights of translation, reprinting, reuse of illustrations, recitation, broadcasting, reproduction on microfilms or in other ways, and storage in data banks.
The use of registered names, trademarks, etc. in this publication does not imply, even in the absence of a specific statement, that such names are exempt from the relevant protective laws and regulations and therefore free for general use.
Product liability: The publisher can give no guarantee for information about drug dosage and application thereof contained in this book. In every individual case the respective user must check its accuracy by consulting other pharmaceutical literature.

Typesetting: Best-set Typesetter Ltd., Hong Kong

SPIN: 10688282

Preface

For more than a decade, the two editors of this book have met annually at the International Scientific Sessions of either the American College of Chest Physicians or the American Heart Association. At these meetings, original research papers from Japan on topics related to pulmonary embolism or deep venous thrombosis were presented. Following these presentations, we began a tradition of meeting informally to compare our experiences as physician-investigators, because we shared a special interest in venous thromboembolism. We always were fascinated by the similar challenges that we faced despite the many contrasts between Asian and Western cultures.

When we first met, we discussed the possibility of undertaking an International Symposium on Pulmonary Embolism. We both felt that such a symposium would improve our understanding of the epidemiology of pulmonary embolism as well as optimize its diagnosis, treatment, and prevention. For two years, we actively organized this symposium, which took place in Mie, Japan, in April 1998 and which was highly successful by all criteria. Subsequently, we decided that a book authored by the international faculty would provide an important educational service to clinicians who care for patients with pulmonary embolism and investigators who research it.

Our objective in *Pulmonary Embolism* is to provide a contemporary overview of the most important issues in pulmonary embolism from a Western and a Japanese perspective. *Pulmonary Embolism* updates various clinical, pathological, and physiological aspects of pulmonary embolism, with separate sections on Hypercoagulability, Diagnosis, Management, and Prevention.

In the Hypercoagulability section, Dr. Ridker presents the state of the art concerning epidemiology, and Dr. Ido elucidates molecular biology that pertains to this illness. The Diagnosis section focuses on optimal strategies to detect venous thromboembolism. Furthermore, in this section, Dr. Ohgi presents a controversial finding—that soleal vein thrombosis, especially when bilateral, is often associated with pulmonary embolism. Dr. Solomon presents exciting new findings concerning echocardiography, and Dr. Yamada illustrates the advantages of magnetic resonance imaging.

The Management section emphasizes an aggressive surgical approach. Dr. Sors provides a Western perspective and Dr. Masuda a Japanese perspective on surgical embolectomy for pulmonary embolism. The nuances of pulmonary thromboendarterectomy are elucidated by Drs. Yutani, Ohteki, and Daily.

The final section of *Pulmonary Embolism* emphasizes the importance of primary and secondary prevention of this potentially devastating illness. Dr. Elliott updates the pharmacological approach with low molecular weight heparins, and Dr. Greenfield, the "Dean" of vena caval interruption, places in perspective the indications for inferior vena caval placement.

We believe our book will be of interest to students, practicing physicians, researchers, and academicians who wish to gain a "cutting edge" viewpoint on key fundamental and clinical issues. Special thanks are due to Naoto Hiraoka, M.D., of the First Department of Internal Medicine at Mie University School of Medicine. Dr. Hiraoka coordinated many of the activities that were essential to the successful publication of this book. The editorial planning and production staff of Springer-Verlag, Tokyo served us with great expertise. Finally, the Goldhaber and Nakano families are credited with patience and understanding while we attended to our important responsibility as Editors.

Samuel Z. Goldhaber
Takeshi Nakano
THE EDITORS

Contents

Management

Prevention

Contributors

Overview

Overview of Pulmonary Embolism

SAMUEL Z. GOLDHABER

Summary. For too long, Eastern and Western cultures have approached the epidemiology, diagnosis, therapy, and prevention of pulmonary embolism in cultural isolation. Although the discovery of the factor V Leiden genetic mutation has revolutionized the epidemiology of venous thromboembolism in Caucasian populations of European ancestry, this finding has not advanced the epidemiological approach to pulmonary embolism in Japan, because this genetic mutation is so rare in Asians. However, advances in reliable noninvasive diagnostic techniques have been welcomed in the East and the West, particularly the D-dimer ELISA, echocardiography, spiral chest CT scanning, and magnetic resonance imaging. The use of subcutaneously administered low molecular weight heparins has made home treatment possible for pulmonary embolism patients at low risk. Perhaps the most exciting advance in therapy is implementation of routine risk stratification, especially by establishing the status of the right ventricle. Right ventricular hypokinesis on echocardiography is becoming increasingly recognized as a poor prognostic sign. By understanding that pulmonary embolism encompasses a wide clinical spectrum, those patients at high risk of an adverse outcome can be selected for thrombolysis or catheter-based or surgical embolectomy in addition to anticoagulation. Finally, prevention of venous thromboembolism is crucially important. While effective pharmacologic strategies can be implemented, especially with low molecular weight heparins, mechanical measures such as insertion of an inferior vena caval filter are also effective.

Keywords. Pulmonary embolism, Venous thromboembolism, Thrombosis, Anticoagulation, Thrombolysis

Cardiovascular Division, Brigham and Women's Hospital, Harvard Medical School, 75 Francis Street, Boston, MA 02115, USA

Introduction

Pulmonary embolism (PE) continues to challenge our clinical skills, despite recent, far-reaching advances (Table 1) in epidemiology, diagnosis, therapy, and prevention. Our International Symposium in Mie, Japan, has provided a unique opportunity for mutual education, collaboration, and scientific interchange. For far too long, Eastern and Western cultures have approached PE in cultural isolation. More than two decades ago, I was taught that PE is virtually exclusively a disease of the Western world. Imagine my surprise when I learned in 1988 that Professor Nakano's Department of Medicine in Mie, Japan, specializes in clinical research and management of PE! In this overview, I present a Western perspective on PE with the hope that our next Symposium will facilitate a more globalized approach to this perplexing and often frustrating medical illness.

Epidemiologically, identification of the autosomal dominant factor V Leiden single amino acid point mutation (adenine for guanine) has permitted detection of families at high risk for development of venous thrombosis [1–3]. In the United States, this mutation in the gene coding for factor V is found in Caucasian-American PE patients far more often than in Asian-Americans [4]. The factor V Leiden mutation results in resistance to activated protein C (APC), a potent endogenous anticoagulant that prolongs the activated partial thromboplastin time (PTT) when added to plasma. Glutamine replaces arginine at position 506, thereby making factor V more difficult for APC to cleave and inactivate.

New diagnostic approaches, particularly plasma D-dimer enzyme-linked immunosorbent assay (ELISA) [5], echocardiography [6], and spiral chest computed tomography (CT) scanning [7, 8], in combination with standard venous ultrasonography [9], have decreased our reliance upon lung scans for routine imaging and on pulmonary angiograms for resolution of diagnostic dilemmas. Thus, reliable, noninvasive diagnosis or exclusion of PE is usually possible if these tests are available and properly utilized.

TABLE 1. Advances in pulmonary embolism (PE)

Category	Advance
Epidemiology	Elucidation of the factor V Leiden mutation and of hyperhomocysteinemia as PE risk factors
Diagnosis	Increased utilization of echocardiography and plasma D-dimer ELISA; decreased reliance upon arterial blood gases
Therapy	Risk stratification of patients, often with echocardiography Low molecular weight heparins Thrombolysis or embolectomy in high-risk patients (even in absence of cardiogenic shock)
Prevention	Low molecular weight heparins Extension of prophylaxis beyond date of hospital discharge

ELISA, enzyme-linked immunosorbent assay.

TABLE 2. Unsolved problems in pulmonary embolism

Category	Unsolved problem
Epidemiology	Persistent high mortality rate Utility of factor V Leiden screening in clinical practice
Diagnosis	Lack of a standard diagnostic approach Critical dependence upon individual physicians to interpret diagnostic tests such as lung scans, echocardiograms, and spiral chest CT scans
Therapy	Lack of consensus on utilizing thrombolysis and embolectomy, especially among PE patients with normal systemic arterial pressure and right ventricular dysfunction
Prevention	Failure to prevent venous thromboembolism among some hospitalized patients despite conscientious implementation Uncertainty regarding optimal regimens for medical patients

CT, computed tomography.

More widespread use of low molecular weight heparins is facilitating the therapeutic objective of rapidly obtaining reliable and effective levels of anticoagulation [10]. These heparins reduce markedly the need for laboratory monitoring and hold promise for shortening the duration of hospitalization among PE patients at low risk. In large, controlled trials, low molecular weight heparins have proved to be as effective and safe as unfractionated heparin for management of both deep venous thrombosis (DVT) [11, 12] and PE [13, 14].

Although anticoagulation remains the foundation of management, some PE patients are at such high risk that additional intervention such as thrombolysis or embolectomy is warranted. It used to be common to risk stratify and prognosticate merely upon the basis of the systemic arterial pressure and heart rate. PE patients who presented with systemic arterial hypotension that did not respond to vasopressor agents were rightfully considered to be at high risk and to have a poor prognosis. Often, they were referred for aggressive intervention after cardiogenic shock had ensued. Under these circumstances, adverse outcomes were inevitably frequent, regardless of therapy. In the new millennium, our ability to risk stratify PE patients has become more sophisticated. Specifically, we now search for signs of right ventricular dysfunction to detect patients with impending hemodynamic instability [15]. Often, PE patients are evaluated with echocardiography so that those with moderate or severe right ventricular dysfunction, even in the presence of normal systemic arterial pressure, can be quickly identified.

Prevention of PE is receiving renewed interest, largely because of the increasing availability of low molecular weight heparins which often appear to provide superior protection than conventional low-dose heparin without an increased risk of bleeding. As hospital stays shorten, prophylaxis is increasingly prescribed for extended durations beyond the hospital discharge date.

Despite these encouraging advances, many clinical problems remain unsolved (Table 2). Death and rehospitalization rates remain high for PE patients. ICOPER, the International Cooperative Pulmonary Embolism Registry, recorded a 3-month mortality rate of 17.5% [16]. At Brigham and Women's Hospital, we recently noted a disturbing clustering of autopsy proven cases of fatal PE.

Although our knowledge of the factor V Leiden mutation has introduced molecular genetics to PE, we do not know how to best use this information and whether screening for the factor V Leiden mutation is worthwhile [17]. On the other hand, we have learned that the presence of the Leiden mutation doubles or triples the risk of recurrent PE after anticoagulation has been discontinued [18, 19].

Diagnostic approaches have not been standardized. Too often, the work-up for PE varies among institutions because of dependence upon an individual physician who is especially skilled in performing and interpreting lung scans, echocardiography, or spiral chest CT scans. Therapeutic approaches also vary. No consensus exists on optimal management of patients with normal systemic arterial pressure and concomitant right ventricular dysfunction. Finally, venous thromboembolism continues to occur de novo in hospitalized patients despite implementation of optimal prophylaxis regimens. Whereas substantial progress has been made in prophylaxis of patients undergoing hip or knee replacement surgery, prevention of PE among medical patients, especially medical Intensive Care Unit patients [20], has not been studied adequately [21].

Pathophysiology

Venous thrombi form in the deep leg and pelvic veins as well as the large upper extremity veins due to an underlying predisposition to hypercoagulability, venous stasis, or trauma. While these thrombi often have no clinical manifestations, they may cause discomfort and swelling. At times, they continue to propagate and eventually embolize to the pulmonary arteries, via the vena cava, right atrium, and right ventricle. Rarely, echocardiography documents "thrombi in transit." The clinical spectrum and pathophysiologic manifestations of PE range from small, incidental thrombosis to massive PE associated with sudden death due to cardiogenic shock. Pulmonary arterial obstruction and platelet secretion of vasoactive agents elevate pulmonary vascular resistance. Increased alveolar dead space impairs gas exchange, and stimulation of irritant receptors causes alveolar hyperventilation. Reflex bronchoconstriction augments airway resistance, and lung edema decreases pulmonary compliance [22]. Elevation in right ventricular pressure can cause an increase in right ventricular wall tension with consequent right ventricular dilatation, dysfunction, and ischemia.

Epidemiology

Incidence

The incidence of venous thromboembolism in the United States is approximately 1 in 1000 per year [23]. More than 250 000 patients are hospitalized annually in the United States with PE or deep venous thrombosis (DVT). One-third of patients suffer recurrent episodes. For each 10-year increase in age, the incidence of venous thrombosis doubles.

Mortality

ICOPER is the largest prospective PE registry ever undertaken, with 2454 consecutive hospitalized PE patients enrolled in 52 participating hospitals from seven Western countries: Italy, the United States, France, Mexico, Switzerland, Poland, and Belguim [16]. Even more surprising than the high 17.5% mortality rate at 3 months follow-up was that PE itself, not cancer, was the principal cause of death.

Risk Factors for Death from Pulmonary Embolism

Right Ventricular Dysfunction

Four PE registries have reported an association between right ventricular dysfunction and adverse clinical outcomes such as death and recurrent PE [16, 24–26]. Although fewer than 5% of ICOPER patients presented in cardiogenic shock, right ventricular hypokinesis as assessed by echocardiography occurred in about 40% of patients with normal systemic arterial pressure. Right ventricular hypokinesis was associated with a doubling of the mortality rate at 14 days and with a 1.5 times higher mortality rate at 3 months [16]. Multivariable analysis showed that right ventricular dysfunction on echocardiography contributed independently to a doubling of the risk of mortality within 3 months.

In a Swedish registry, 126 consecutive PE patients underwent echocardiography when PE was initially diagnosed [24]. The overall 1-year mortality rate was 15%. However, among those with right ventricular dysfunction, the mortality rate at 1 year was threefold higher than for patients with normal right ventricular function (Fig. 1). Similar findings were reported in Kasper's PE registry of

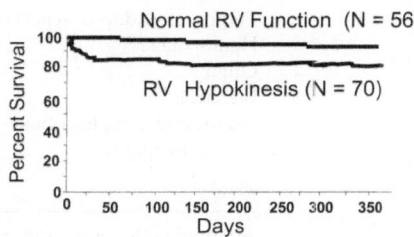

FIG. 1. One-year survival in pulmonary embolism patients with normal and depressed right ventricular function on echocardiography. (From [24], with permission)

317 patients [25]. Finally, the large *M*anagement Strategy *A*nd *P*rognosis of *P*ulmonary *E*mbolism Regis*t*ry (MAPPET) enrolled 1001 patients with PE and right ventricular dysfunction [26]. As right heart failure worsened, the mortality rate increased.

Risk Factors for Developing Pulmonary Embolism

Genetic predisposition explains only a minority of PE cases. Therefore, identification of potentially modifiable risk factors is critical. In the Nurses' Health Study [27], the highest rates of PE were observed among nurses 60 years of age or older who were obese. Because obesity is a much more pervasive problem in Western compared with Eastern societies, the higher prevalence of obesity in the West may correlate with higher Western rates of PE. In the Nurses' Health Study, heavy cigarette smoking and high blood pressure were also identified as risk factors for PE. However, no association was observed with high cholesterol or diabetes.

Pregnancy and Oral Contraceptives

For women whose pregnancies resulted in a live birth, thrombotic PE was the leading cause of death [28] (Table 3). Oral contraceptives (OCs) triple the risk of venous thromboembolism in users compared with nonusers. Although the relative risk is high, the absolute risk is low and estimated at about one additional PE or DVT per 10 000 person-years. "Third-generation OCs" contain desogestrel, gestodene, or norgestimate as the progesterone (in combination with low-dose estrogen) and appear to be especially thrombogenic, and attenuate the androgenic side effects of acne and hirsutism [29–31]. These unexpected observations have provided a new appreciation of the thrombogenicity of progesterones.

Postmenopausal Hormone Replacement Therapy

For the past generation, use of postmenopausal estrogens was not considered to increase the risk of venous thromboembolism. The rationale was

TABLE 3. Causes of maternal death among pregnancies resulting in live birth, United States, 1979–1986

Cause of death	Number (%)
Pulmonary embolism	370 (27.1%)
Pregnancy-induced hypertension	307 (22.5%)
Hemorrhage	249 (18.3%)
Other	218 (16.0%)
Infection	101 (7.4%)
Anesthesia complications	65 (4.8%)
Cardiomyopathy	53 (3.9%)
Total	1363 (100%)

Adapted with permission from [28].

that the estrogen content of postmenopausal hormones is trivial compared with that of OCs. However, data from three recent studies indicate that hormone replacement therapy doubles the risk of venous thromboembolism [32–34]. The risk is higher near the start of therapy than after chronic use.

Surgery

Surgery predisposes to PE, and this susceptibility persists for up to 1 month postoperatively [35, 36]. Thus, the risk of delayed postoperative PE must be considered when devising optimal strategies to prevent venous thromboembolism.

Cancer

Occasionally, previously unsuspected cancer will be diagnosed in patients with newly established venous thrombosis [37]. Adenocarcinomas of breast, pancreas, ovary, and lung are most commonly associated with PE. The suspected mechanism is generation of thrombin and secretion of procoagulants by neoplastic cells [38].

Factor V Leiden

In the Physicians' Health Study [3], the relative risk of venous thrombosis was 2.7 if the factor V Leiden mutation was present. Using the Physicians' Health Study database [39], factor V Leiden was eightfold more common in men with venous thrombosis who were older than age 70 compared with those younger than age 50.

Hyperhomocysteinemia

There is a 2–3-fold increased risk of DVT in patients with plasma hyperhomocysteinemia [40, 41]. In the Physicians' Health Study [42], hyperhomocysteinemia tripled the risk of idiopathic venous thrombosis, and factor V Leiden doubled the risk of venous thrombosis. However, combined hyperhomocysteinemia and factor V Leiden increased the risk almost tenfold.

Antiphospholipid Antibody Syndrome and Lupus Anticoagulant

This acquired abnormality may be associated with an increased risk of venous thrombosis, recurrent spontaneous miscarriage, stroke, or pulmonary hypertension [43].

Deficiencies of Endogenous Coagulation Proteins

Since deficiencies of antithrombin III, protein C, and protein S are rare, they should not be sought during the routine work-up for hypercoagulability. In one western European cohort with venous thrombosis, antithrombin III deficiency was identified in 1% of patients, and protein C or S deficiencies were identified in 3% and 2%, respectively [44].

Diagnosis

PE, known as the "great masquerader," can accompany or mimic other cardiopulmonary illnesses. Its differential diagnosis is extensive (Table 4). Whereas dyspnea, syncope, or cyanosis usually indicate a massive PE, pleuritic pain, cough, or hemoptysis often suggest a small embolism located distally near the pleura. Many patients with massive PE preserve adequate systemic arterial pressure until immediately before their demise. Their physical findings may include: bulging neck veins with v waves, a left parasternal lift, an accentuated pulmonic component of the second heart sound, and a systolic murmur at the left lower sternal border that increases in intensity during inspiration.

The most frequent electrocardiographic abnormality is T-wave inversion in the anterior chest leads, V1–V4 [45]. A pattern of S in lead I, Q in lead III, and T-wave inversion in lead III is rarely seen but is associated with PE. New-onset right bundle branch block or atrial fibrillation is far less common. Although the chest X-ray is often normal, specific findings may include: focal oligemia (Westermark's sign), a peripheral wedge-shaped density above the diaphragm (Hampton's hump), or an enlarged right descending pulmonary artery (Palla's sign).

Arterial blood gases cannot accurately discriminate between those patients suspected of PE who require further investigation and those in whom no further work-up is required [46, 47]. However, the plasma D-dimer ELISA may be a useful screening test because even with PE, there is usually some endogenous

TABLE 4. Differential diagnosis

Pneumonia, asthma, COPD exacerbation, bronchitis, or lung cancer
Myocardial infarction
Costochondritis, "viral syndrome," or anxiety
Dissection of the aorta
Pericardial tamponade
Lung cancer
Primary pulmonary hypertension
Rib fracture or pneumothorax
Musculoskeletal pain

COPD, chronic obstructive pulmonary disease.

(although clinically ineffective) fibrinolysis. When plasmin digests cross-linked fibrin from the PE that has formed, D-dimers are released into the plasma and can be recognized by commercially available monoclonal antibodies. A D-dimer ELISA >500 ng/ml is abnormal and is present in more than 90% of patients with PE. Conversely, a normal D-dimer ELISA provides reassurance in more than 90% of cases that PE is not present. Unfortunately, the D-dimer ELISA lacks specificity and is elevated in patients with myocardial infarction, pneumonia, heart failure, cancer, and following surgery. Therefore, this test is most useful when used to screen patients who present to the Emergency Department or office without other systemic illness [48].

Although the presence of DVT can generally be used as a surrogate for PE, a major caveat is that a normal leg-imaging test cannot exclude PE if clinical suspicion is moderately high. In a series of 41 PE patients who underwent both pulmonary angiography and bilateral contrast venography of the legs, 12 had negative leg venograms despite positive pulmonary angiograms [49].

Unfortunately, even the high-probability lung scan is surprisingly insensitive and in PIOPED, it identified only 41% of patients with PE [50]. In the majority of patients with PE, the lung scan is, regrettably, nondiagnostic despite complex revisions of PIOPED diagnostic criteria [51]. Ventilation scanning rarely clarifies the interpretation of perfusion lung scans [52]. Furthermore, in the presence of high clinical suspicion for PE, the "low probability" lung scan is a potentially lethal reading [53], which is more accurately categoried as "nondiagnostic" [54]. The problem is that the term "low probability" can convey a false sense of security to the physician.

Spiral chest CT scanning with contrast is a new diagnostic approach best suited for identifying PE in the proximal pulmonary vascular tree [55]. Another promising new technology is gadolinium-enhanced magnetic resonance pulmonary angiography [56], which can display the anatomy of the pulmonary arteries as well as provide an assessment of right ventricular wall motion.

Transthoracic echocardiography is particularly useful in critically ill patients with suspected PE [57] and can help identify conditions which mimic PE such as myocardial infarction, dissection of the aorta, or pericardial tamponade. The thrombus itself is rarely visualized. Signs of right ventricular pressure overload include: right ventricular dilatation, right ventricular hypokinesis, pulmonary arterial hypertension as assessed by Doppler, interventricular septal flattening and displacement into the left ventricle, and impaired left ventricular relaxation with a D-shaped left ventricle in cross section. Detection of right ventricular hypertrophy suggests that the process is chronic, subacute, or acute superimposed upon chronic. The McConnell sign may be specific for acute PE and is defined as a pattern of regional right ventricular dysfunction in which right ventricular apical wall motion remains normal despite hypokinesis of the right ventricular free wall. A "hinge point" is observed at the border of the mid apical free wall and the apex [58].

Contrast pulmonary angiography remains the gold standard. It can generally be performed safely [59] and may resolve the dilemma of high clinical suspicion despite nondiagnostic lung scanning, normal venous ultrasonography, and normal echocardiography.

Therapy

Heparin accelerates the action of antithrombin III, prevents additional thrombus from forming, and promotes endothelialization of clot. Patients suspected of PE should be expeditiously and intensively anticoagulated with heparin while definitive diagnostic testing is under way. A bolus (average 7500 units) followed by a continuous infusion of unfractionated heparin (average 1250 units/h), usually achieves rapidly a therapeutic activated partial thromboplastin time (PTT) between 60 and 80 s. Nomograms facilitate proper dosing and adjustment of the heparin concentration [60]. Rapid achievement of a therapeutic heparin level minimizes the likelihood of recurrent PE [61]. Heparin without oral anticoagulation is used throughout pregnancy to manage PE [62]. Heparin is also employed in Trousseau's syndrome for both acute and chronic therapy, because oral anticoagulation usually fails to prevent recurrent thrombosis [63]. Recently, inpatient administration of low molecular weight heparin has received FOA approval because it has been shown to be as safe and effective as unfractionated heparin to treat hemodynamically stable PE [64, 65].

Inferior vena caval (IVC) filters appear to offer no advantage compared with anticoagulation alone in patients with free-floating proximal DVT [66]. Filters do not halt the thrombotic process and may cause massive leg edema due to caval thrombosis. In a randomized controlled trial of 400 DVT patients, IVC filters plus anticoagulation did not reduce mortality compared with anticoagulation alone [67]. However, an IVC filter is indicated for PE patients who present with active hemorrhage or recurrent PE despite intensive and prolonged anticoagulation.

Warfarin can be safely started immediately after obtaining a therapeutic PTT or heparin level. Loading warfarin does not shorten the usual 5 days needed to achieve adequate oral anticoagulation. An initial average dose of 5 mg usually suffices [68], except for small, debilitated, or elderly patients in whom a 2 mg dose is prudent, or large, young, otherwise healthy patients in whom a 7.5 mg dose is reasonable. Although 2.0–3.0 is usually considered the target international normalized ratio (INR), an INR of 3.0 is ideal in patients without additional risk factors for bleeding complications. Recently, the use of concomitant acetaminophen and warfarin has been detected as a common cause of overanticoagulation in the outpatient setting [69].

After an initial PE, 6 months of anticoagulation prevents far more recurrences than 6 weeks [70]. Indefinite anticoagulation should be considered in patients with recurrent PE if their risk of major bleeding is low [71]. Whether patients with factor V Leiden and an initial PE should receive prolonged courses of anticoagulation remains sharply debated.

Although there is consensus that thrombolysis can be lifesaving in patients with massive PE, controversy persists regarding its use in PE patients with stable systemic arterial pressure and right ventricular dysfunction. A randomized controlled trial [72] and multivariate analysis of a large German registry [73] suggest that in patients with right ventricular dysfunction, thrombolysis may lower the rate of recurrent PE compared with heparin alone. However, the risk of major hemorrhage rises with increasing age and body mass index [74]. If aggressive intervention is warranted in the setting of failed or contraindicated thrombolysis, transvenous catheter [75] or open surgical embolectomy [76] should be considered.

Prevention

Although no prophylaxis method is perfect, virtually all hospitalized patients at moderate or high risk should receive mechanical or pharmacological prophylaxis. Mechanical methods include graduated compression stockings (GCS), intermittent pneumatic compression (IPC) devices, or IVC filters. Foot pumps are also available for prophylaxis, but they have not been extensively investigated in rigorous clinical trials.

Pharmacologic methods include fixed low-dose subcutaneous unfractionated heparin ("miniheparin"), low molecular weight heparin, and warfarin. Miniheparin reduces the perioperative rate of fatal PE by two-thirds [77]. The typical dose is 5000 units twice or three times daily. An initial injection is administered 2 h before the skin incision, and miniheparin is continued until the patient is discharged and fully ambulatory.

Low molecular weight heparins have superior bioavailability, require less frequent injections, and have reduced rates of heparin-induced thrombocytopenia than miniheparin [78]. Currently, three low molecular weight heparins—enoxaparin, dalteparin, and ardeparin—and one heparinoid, danaparoid [79], have received Food and Drug Administration approval for specific prophylaxis indications. Table 5 lists various prophylaxis strategies.

Conclusions

The epidemiology, diagnosis, treatment, and prophylaxis of PE are rapidly advancing. There is now an increased understanding of inherited and environmental risks. Our diagnostic armamentarium has expanded to include the plasma D-dimer ELISA, echocardiography, spiral chest CT with contrast, and magnetic resonance imaging. We have also gained a keen appreciation for the importance of risk stratification based upon right ventricular function when PE is initially detected. The availability of low molecular weight heparins has broadened our options both for treatment and for prophylaxis. As the new millennium approaches, our task will be to develop and implement a

TABLE 5. Prevention of venous thromboembolism

Condition	Prophylaxis strategy
General surgery	UFH 5000 U BID/TID or Enoxaparin 40 mg SC q 24 h or Dalteparin 2500 or 5000 U SC q 24 h
Total hip replacement	Warfarin (target INR 2.5) or IPC or Enoxaparin 30 mg SC BID or Danaparoid 750 U SC BID
Total knee replacement	Enoxaparin 30 mg SC BID or Ardeparin 50 U/kg SC BID
General medical patient	GCS or IPC or UFH 5000 U BID/TID

GCS, graduated compression stockings; UFH, unfractionated heparin; IPC, intermittent pneumatic compression device; INR, international normalized ratio.

global strategy that is tailored for adaptability in both Western and Eastern populations.

References

1. Svensson PJ, Dahlbäck B (1994) Resistance to activated protein C as a basis for venous thrombosis. New Engl J Med 330:517–522
2. Bertina RM, Koeleman BPC, Koster T et al. (1994) Mutation in blood coagulation factor V associated with resistance to activated protein C. Nature 369:64–67
3. Ridker PM, Hennekens CH, Lindpaintner K (1995) Mutation in the gene coding for coagulation factor V and risks of future myocardial infarction, stroke, and venous thrombosis in apparently healthy men. N Engl J Med 332:912–917
4. Ridker PM, Miletich JP, Hennekens CH, Buring JE (1997) Ethnic distribution of factor V Leiden in 4047 men and women. Implications for venous thromboembolism screening. JAMA 277:1305–1307
5. Bounameaux H, de Moerloose P, Perrier A, Miron MJ (1997) D-dimer testing in suspected venous thromboembolism: an update. Q J Med 90:437–442
6. Jardin F, Dubourg O, Bourdarias JP (1997) Echocardiographic pattern of acute cor pulmonale. Chest 111:209–217
7. Remy-Jardin M, Remy J, Deschildre F et al. (1996) Diagnosis of pulmonary embolism with spiral CT: comparison with pulmonary angiography and scintigraphy. Radiology 200:699–706
8. Goodman LR, Lipchik RJ (1996) Diagnosis of acute pulmonary embolism: time for a new approach. Radiology 199:25–27
9. Lensing AWA, Prandoni P, Brandjes D et al. (1989) Detection of deep-vein thrombosis by real-time B-mode ultrasonography. N Engl J Med 320:342–345
10. Weitz JI (1997) Low-molecular-weight heparins. N Engl J Med 337:688–698
11. Koopman MMW, Prandoni P, Piovella F et al. (1996) Treatment of venous thrombosis with intravenous unfractionated heparin administered in the hospital as compared

with subcutaneous low-molecular-weight heparin administered at home. N Engl J Med 334:682–687

12. Levine M, Gent M, Hirsh J et al. (1996) A comparison of low-molecular-weight heparin administered primarily at home with unfractionated heparin administered in the hospital for proximal deep-vein thrombosis. N Engl J Med 334:677–681

13. The Columbus Investigators (1997) Low-molecular-weight heparin in the treatment of patients with venous thromboembolism. N Engl J Med 337:657–662

14. Simonneau G, Sors H, Charbonnier B et al. (1997) A comparison of low-molecular-weight-heparin with unfractionated heparin for acute pulmonary embolism. N Engl J Med 337:663–669

15. Cannon CP, Goldhaber SZ (1995) The importance of rapidly treating patients with acute myocardial infarction. Chest 107:598–600

16. Goldhaber SZ, Visani L, De Rosa M (1999) Acute pulmonary embolism: clinical outcomes in the International Cooperative Pulmonary Embolism Registry Lancet. (in press)

17. Price DT, Ridker PM (1997) Factor V Leiden mutation and the risks for thromboembolic disease: a clinical perspective. Ann Intern Med 127:895–903

18. Simioni P, Prandoni P, Lensing AWA et al. (1997) The risk of recurrent venous thromboembolism in patients with an Arg^{506} → Gln mutation in the gene for factor V (factor V Leiden). N Engl J Med 336:399–403

19. Ridker PM, Miletich JP, Stampfer MJ et al. (1995) Factor V Leiden and risks of recurrent idiopathic venous thromboembolism. Circulation 92:2800–2802

20. Hirsch DR, Ingenito EP, Goldhaber SZ (1995) Prevalence of deep venous thrombosis among patients in medical intensive care. JAMA 274:335–337

21. Goldhaber SZ (1998) Venous thromboembolism in the Intensive Care Unit: the last frontier for prophylaxis. Chest 113:5–7

22. Elliott CG (1992) Pulmonary physiology during pulmonary embolism. Chest 101:163S–171S

23. Anderson FA Jr, Wheeler HB, Goldberg RJ et al. (1991) A population-based perspective of the hospital incidence and case-fatality rates of venous thrombosis and pulmonary embolism: The Worcester DVT Study. Arch Intern Med 151:933–938

24. Ribeiro A, Lindmarker P, Juhlin-Dannfelt A, Johnsson H, Jorfeldt L (1997) Echocardiography Doppler in pulmonary embolism: right ventricular dysfunction as predictor of mortality. Am Heart J 134:479–487

25. Kasper W, Konstantinides S, Geibel A et al. (1997) Prognostic significance of right ventricular afterload stress detected by echocardiography in patients with clinically suspected pulmonary embolism. Heart 77:346–349

26. Kasper W, Konstantinides S, Geibel A et al. (1997) Management strategies and determinants of outcome in acute major pulmonary embolism: results of a multicenter registry. J Am Coll Cardiol 30:1165–1171

27. Goldhaber SZ, Grodstein F, Stampfer MJ et al. (1997) A prospective study of risk factors for pulmonary embolism in women. JAMA 277:642–645

28. Koonin LM, Atrash HK, Lawson HW, Smith JC (1991) Maternal Mortality Surveillance, United States, 1979–1986. CDC Surveillance Summaries. MMWR 40:1–8

29. World Health Organization Collaborative Study of Cardiovascular Disease and Steroid Hormone Contraception (1995) Venous thromboembolic disease and combined oral contraceptives: results of international multicentre case-control study. Lancet 346:1575–1582

30. World Health Organization Collaborative Study of Cardiovascular Disease and Steroid Hormone Contraception (1995) Effect of different progestagens in low oestrogen oral contraceptives on venous thromboembolic disease. Lancet 346:1582–1588

31. Jick H, Jick SS, Gurewich V, Myers MW, Vasilakis C (1995) Risk of idiopathic cardiovascular death and nonfatal venous thromboembolism in women using oral contraceptives with differing progestagen components. Lancet 346:1589–1593

32. Daly E, Vessey MP, Hawkins MM (1996) Risk of venous thromboembolism in users of hormone replacement therapy. Lancet 348:977–980

33. Jick H, Derby LE, Myers MW, Vasilakis C, Newton KM (1996) Risk of hospital admission for idiopathic venous thromboembolism among users of postmenopausal oestrogens. Lancet 348:981–983

34. Grodstein F, Stampfer MJ, Goldhaber SZ (1996) Prospective study of exogenous hormones and risk of pulmonary embolism in women. Lancet 348:983–987

35. Bergqvist D, Lindblad B (1985) A 30-year survey of pulmonary embolism verified at autopsy: an analysis of 1274 surgical patients. Br J Surg 72:105–108

36. Huber O, Bounameaux H, Borst F, Rohner A (1992) Postoperative pulmonary embolism after hospital discharge. An underestimated risk. Arch Surg 127:310–313

37. Prandoni P, Lensing AWA, Büller HR et al. (1992) Deep vein thrombosis and the incidence of subsequent symptomatic cancer. N Engl J Med 327:1128–1133

38. Piccioli A, Prandoni P, Ewenstein BM, Goldhaber SZ (1996) Cancer and venous thromboembolism. Am Heart J 132:850–855

39. Ridker PM, Glynn RJ, Miletich JP et al. (1997) Age-specific incidence rates of venous thromboembolism among heterozygous carriers of factor V Leiden mutation. Ann Intern Med 126:528–531

40. Simioni P, Prandoni P, Burlina A et al. (1996) Hyperhomocysteinemia and deep-vein thrombosis. A case control study. Thromb Haemost 76:883–886

41. den Heijer M, Koster T, Blom HJ (1996) Hyperhomocysteinemia as a risk factor for deep-vein thrombosis. N Engl J Med 334:759–762

42. Ridker PM, Hennekens CH, Selhub J et al. (1997) Interrelation of hyperhomocyst(e)inemia, factor V Leiden, and risk of future venous thromboembolism. Circulation 95:1777–1782

43. Hughes GRV (1993) The antiphospholipid syndrome: ten years on. Lancet 342:341–344

44. Heijboer H, Brandjes DPM, Büller HR, Sturk A, ten Cate JW (1990) Deficiencies of coagulation-inhibiting and fibrinolytic proteins in outpatients with deep-vein thrombosis. N Engl J Med 323:1512–1516

45. Ferrari E, Imbert A, Chevalier T et al. (1997) The ECG in pulmonary embolism. Predictive value of negative T waves in precordial leads—80 case reports. Chest 111:537–543

46. Stein PD, Goldhaber SZ, Henry JW, Miller AC (1996) Arterial blood gas analysis in the assessment of suspected acute pulmonary embolism. Chest 109:78–81

47. Stein, PD, Goldhaber SZ, Henry JW (1995) Alveolar-arterial oxygen gradient in the assessment of acute pulmonary embolism. Chest 107:139–143

48. Bounameaux H, de Moerloose P, Perrier A, Miron MJ (1997) D-dimer testing in suspected venous thromboembolism: an update. Q J Med 90:437–442

49. Hull RD, Hirsh J, Carter CJ et al. (1983) Pulmonary angiography, ventilation lung scanning, and venography for clinically suspected pulmonary embolism with abnormal perfusion lung scan. Ann Intern Med 98:891–899

50. PIOPED Investigators (1990) Value of the ventilation perfusion scan in acute pulmonary embolism. Results of the prospective investigation of pulmonary embolism diagnosis (PIOPED). JAMA 263: 2753–2759
51. Gottschalk A, Sostman HD, Coleman RE et al. (1993) Ventilation-perfusion scintigraphy in the PIOPED study. Part II. Evaluation of the scintigraphic criteria and interpretations. J Nucl Med 34:1119–1126
52. Stein PD, Terrin ML, Gottschalk A, Alavi A, Henry JW (1992) Value of ventilation/perfusion scans versus perfusion scans alone in acute pulmonary embolism. Am J Cardiol 69:1239–1242
53. Bone RC (1993) The low-probability lung scan. A potentially lethal reading. Arch Intern Med 153:2621–2622
54. Hull RD, Raskob GE, Pineo GF, Brant RF (1995) The low-probability lung scan. A need for change in nomenclature. Arch Intern Med 155:1845–1851
55. Remy-Jardin M, Remy J, Deschildre F et al. (1996) Diagnosis of pulmonary embolism with spiral CT: comparison with pulmonary angiography and scintigraphy. Radiology 200:699–706
56. Meaney JFM, Weg JG, Chenevert TL et al. (1997) Diagnosis of pulmonary embolism with magnetic resonance angiography. N Engl J Med 336:1422–1427
57. Jardin F, Dubourg O, Bourdarias JP (1997) Echocardiographic pattern of acute cor pulmonale. Chest 111:209–217
58. McConnell MV, Solomon SD, Rayan ME et al. (1996) Regional right ventricular dysfunction detected by echocardiography in acute pulmonary embolism (The "hinge point" sign). Am J Cardiol 78:769–473
59. Stein PD, Athanasoulis C, Alavi A et al. (1992) Complications and validity of pulmonary angiography in acute pulmonary embolism. Circulation 85:462–468
60. Raschke RA, Reilly BM, Guidry JR, Fontana JR, Srinivas S (1993) The weight-based heparin dosing nomogram compared with a "standard care" nomogram: a randomized controlled trial. Ann Intern Med 119:874–881
61. Hull RD, Raskob GE, Brant RF, Pineo GF, Valentine KA (1997) Relation between the time to achieve the lower limit of the APTT therapeutic range and recurrent venous thromboembolism during heparin treatment for deep vein thrombosis. Arch Intern Med 157:2562–2568
62. Toglia MR, Weg JG (1996) Venous thromboembolism during pregnancy. N Engl J Med 335:108–114
63. Callander N, Rapaport SI (1993) Trousseau's syndrome. West J Med 158:364–371
64. The COLUMBUS Investigators (1997) Low-molecular-weight heparin in the treatment of patients with venous thromboembolism. N Engl J Med 337:657–662
65. Simonneau G, Sors H, Charbonnier B et al. (1997) A comparison of low-molecular-weight-heparin with unfractionated heparin for acute pulmonary embolism. N Engl J Med 337:663–669
66. Pacouret G, Alison D, Pottier J-M, Bertrand P, Charbonnier B (1997) Free-floating thrombus and embolis risk in patients with angiographically confirmed proximal deep venous thrombosis. A prospective study. Arch Intern Med 157:305–308
67. Decousus H, Leizorovicz A, Parent F et al. (1998) A clinical trial of vena caval filters in the prevention of pulmonary embolism in patients with proximal deep-vein thrombosis. N Engl J Med 338:409–415
68. Harrison L, Johnston M, Massicotte MP, Crowther M, Moffat K, Hirsh J. Comparison of 5-mg and 10-mg loading doses in initiation of warfarin therapy. Ann Intern Med 126:133–136

69. Hylek EM, Heiman H, Skates SJ, Sheehan MA, Singer DE (1998) Acetaminophen and other risk factors for excessive warfarin anticoagulation. JAMA 279:657–662
70. Schulman S, Rhedin A-S, Lindmarker P et al. (1995) A comparison of six weeks with six months of oral anticoagulant therapy after a first episode of venous thromboembolism. N Engl J Med 332:1661–1665
71. Schulman S, Granqvist S, Holmström et al. (1997) The duration of oral anticoagulant therapy after a second episode of venous thromboembolism. N Engl J Med 336:393–398
72. Goldhaber SZ, Haire WD, Feldstein ML et al. (1993) Alteplase versus heparin in acute pulmonary embolism: randomised trial assessing right ventricular function and pulmonary perfusion. Lancet 341:507–511
73. Konstantinides S, Geibel A, Olschewski M et al. (1997) Association between thrombolytic treatment and the prognosis of hemodynamically stable patients with major pulmonary embolism. Results of a multicenter registry. Circulation 96:882–888
74. Mikkola KM, Patel SR, Parker JA, Grodstein F, Goldhaber SZ (1997) Increasing age is a major risk factor for hemorrhagic complications after pulmonary embolism thrombolysis. Am Heart J 134:69–72
75. Greenfield LJ, Proctor MC, Williams DM, Wakefield TW (1993) Long-term experience with transvenous catheter pulmonary embolectomy. J Vasc Surg 18:450–458
76. Gulba DC, Schmid C, Borst H-G et al. (1994) Medical compared with surgical treatment for massive pulmonary embolism. Lancet 343:576–577
77. Collins R, Scrimgeour A, Yusuf S, Peto R (1988) Reduction in fatal pulmonary embolism and venous thrombosis by perioperative administration of subcutaneous heparin. Overview of results of randomized trials in general, orthopedic, and urologic surgery. N Engl J Med 318:1162–1173
78. Weitz JI (1997) Low-molecular-weight heparins. N Engl J Med 337:688–698
79. Hoek JA, Nurmohamed MT, Hamelynck KJ et al. (1992) Prevention of deep vein thrombosis following total hip replacement by low molecular weight heparinoid. Thromb Haemost 67:28–32

Hypercoagulability

Hereditary Thrombophilia Caused by Abnormality of the Anticoagulant Protein C Pathway: Prenatal Diagnosis of Compound Heterozygous Protein C Deficiency by Direct Detection of the Mutation Sites

MASARU IDO, TATSUYA HAYASHI, JUNJI NISHIOKA, and KOJI SUZUKI

Summary. In the present study, we report the molecular characterization of a hereditary compound heterozygous protein C (PC) deficiency observed in a male infant with neonatal purpura fulminans, and its prenatal diagnosis done by direct detection of the mutation sites in the PC gene. DNA-sequence analysis of the patient's and his mother's PC gene disclosed the presence of a deletion of one of the four consecutive G nucleotides encoding $Trp^{380}(TGG)$-$Gly^{381}(GGT)$ in exon IX, resulting in a frameshift mutation, and an abnormal sequence of the 81 amino acid residues following Val^{381}; this mutation was the same as previously reported as PC-Nagoya. The patient's and his father's PC gene had a missense mutation (G to A) in exon III with a substitution of Lys for Glu^{26}; this mutation was named PC-Mie. This mutation may be responsible for the reduced immunological PC levels detected in the patient and the father, as measured by a monoclonal antibody that recognizes the Gla-domain of PC in a Ca^{2+}-dependent manner (3.8% and 57%, respectively). Abnormal PC/activated PC (APC) purified from the father's plasma showed a decreased binding ability to phospholipids, thrombomodulin, and to endothelial cell PC receptor, suggesting that Gla^{26}-dependent conformation is required for these bindings. The proband died at 3 years old. Thereafter, the parents insisted on having a healthy baby. The second pregnancy resulted in spontaneous abortion. During the third and fourth pregnancies, prenatal screening of PC abnormalities was performed. We detected the above-mentioned mutations using two methods; one was based on the development of new restriction enzyme sites using mutagenic primer and the other was the single nucleotide primer extension. In the third pregnancy, the fetus presented both paternal and maternal mutations and thus the pregnancy was ter-

Department of Molecular Pathobiology, Mie University School of Medicine, 174-2-Edobashi, Tsu, Mie 514-8507, Japan

minated by artificial abortion. In the fourth pregnancy, the fetus was free from both mutations, the pregnancy continued, and the woman underwent a cesarean section. The plasma level of Gla-PC antigen in the cord of the female baby was within the normal range. Postnatal analysis of her PC gene disclosed identical results to those done in the prenatal period.

Keywords. Protein C, Hereditary protein C deficiency, Hereditary thrombophilia, Purpura fulminans, Prenatal diagnosis

Introduction

Protein C (PC) is a member of the vitamin K-dependent plasma glycoproteins, which share high amino acid sequence identity [1, 2]. It is fully activated by thrombin bound to thrombomodulin (TM) on the endothelial cell surface [3–5]. To maintain the fluidity of blood, activated PC acts via at least two different mechanisms. First, it exerts an anticoagulant effect by degrading factors Va and VIIIa in concert with protein S [6, 7]. The second antithrombotic action of PC is its stimulatory effect on fibrinolysis by neutralizing plasminogen activator inhibitor-1 [8] or by decreasing the level of thrombin that activates thrombin activable fibrinolysis inhibitor (TAFI) [9]. PC, synthesized in the liver, is composed of a light (22 kDa) and a heavy (40 kDa) chain, linked by a disulfide bond with a molecular weight of 62 kDa [1, 2]. The nucleotide sequence of the PC gene is composed of nine exons (Fig. 1) [10]. These DNA elements code for a leader sequence, a domain containing nine γ-carboxyglutamic acids (Gla-domain), two epidermal growth factor (EGF)-like domains, an activation peptide, and a catalytic domain which is highly homologous in amino acid sequence to other serine proteases. Patients with congenital PC deficiency tend to develop venous thrombosis, such as deep vein thrombosis and pulmonary thromboembolism [11]. So far, two types of PC deficiency (type I and type II) have been reported [12]. In the type I PC deficiency, both the level of PC activity (amidolytic or anticoagulant activity) and the PC antigen level are decreased, the type I thus showing a normal ratio of the

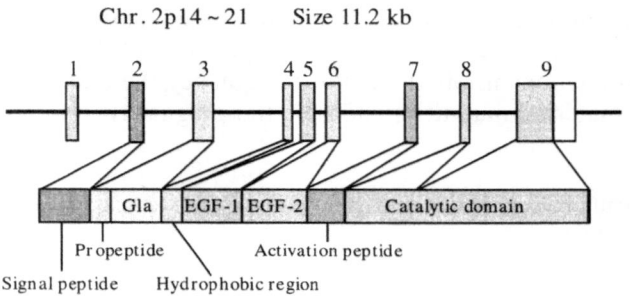

Fig. 1. Structure of protein C gene

activity to the antigen (>0.75). In the type II PC deficiency, the anticoagulant activity of PC is decreased while the PC antigen level remains normal, resulting in a decreased PC activity/PC antigen ratio (<0.75). Homozygous or compound heterozygous PC deficiency is a rare but fatal hereditary condition, characterized by the occurrence of massive disseminated intravascular coagulation (DIC) and neonatal purpura fulminans [4, 5]. In this study we analyzed PC genetic defects in a patient with purpura fulminans. We identified two types of inherited mutations in exons III and IX causing types II and I PC deficiencies, respectively. Furthermore, we characterized the abnormal PC purified from the father's plasma. Based on these results, we performed prenatal screening of these PC gene abnormalities using two methods: (1) single nucleotide primer extension, and (2) development of new restriction enzyme sites in mutant allele by amplifying DNA fragments with mutagenic primers.

Materials and Methods

Family Study

A Japanese male infant was born at term by vaginal delivery on November 16, 1989. At birth, the baby looked well. However, at the age of 1 day, he developed subcutaneous bleeding in the scalp and both soles, intracranial bleeding, and DIC. He was referred to the newborn intensive care unit of our university hospital. Septicemia was initially suspected, but no organism could be identified from blood cultures. After treatment with heparin, fresh frozen plasma, and transfusion for 18 days, his bleeding tendency disappeared. However, 2 days after withdrawal of the treatment, he developed skin bleeding followed by skin necrosis in the scalp and feet, gangrene, and eventual toe amputation. After the recurrence of bleeding, he was treated with fresh frozen plasma and warfarin. At the time of delivery, the mother and father were 32 and 28 years old, respectively. There was no family history of thrombotic disease, bleeding tendency, or consanguinity.

Determination of Plasma Protein C Antigen

Two solid-phase sandwich enzyme-linked immunosorbent assays (ELISAs) were used to determine PC antigen levels. Two monoclonal antibodies recognizing different epitopes in the heavy chain of PC [13, 14] were used to measure total PC antigen. To measure Gla-containing PC, a monoclonal antibody that recognizes the Ca^{2+}-dependent conformation of PC Gla-domain was used as the second fluid-phase antibody (Teijin, Tokyo, Japan) [15].

Determination of Plasma Protein C Activity

The amidolytic and anticoagulant activities of PC after activation with snake venom Protac were determined by using S-2366, Pyro-Glu-Pro-Arg-pNA (Kabi,

Sweden) as a substrate (COATEST protein C) [16] and by measuring prolongation of activated partial thromboplastin time (Protein C reagent Coagulometric, Behring, Germany), respectively.

Purification of Protein C-Mie

PC-Mie was purified from plasma of the patient's father with compound heterozygous PC deficiency; purification of this abnormal PC (APC) was performed using diethylaminoethanol ion exchange HPLC as previously described [17]. The purity of PC-Mie was approximately 90%, as judged from the data obtained by sodium dodecyl sulfate–polyacrylamide gel electrophoresis, a sandwich-type ELISA specific for PC, and a protein concentration assay performed using the Bio-Rad protein assay kit (Bio-Rad, Hercules, CA, USA).

Functional Characterization of Protein C-Mie

Normal PC and APC were compared with PC-Mie and APC-Mie as previously described [18] in terms of following functional characteristics: (1) activation of PC by thrombin and TM or rsTM [19] or on endothelial surface; (2) inactivation of factor Va by APC in the presence of phospholipids; (3) binding of PC or APC to phospholipids, biotinyl-factor Va, or protein S; (4) inhibition of APC by protein C inhibitor (PCI) [20].

Flow Cytometric Analysis of the Binding of Protein C and Abnormal Protein C to Endothelial Cells

Cultured human umbilical endothelial cells (1×10^5 cells) suspended in Hank's balanced salt solution containing 1.3 mM $CaCl_2$, 1% BSA, and 0.002% sodium azide were incubated with PC, APC, Gla-domainless PC, or Gla-domainless APC (78 nM final concentration) at room temperature for 45 min. After washing three times with the same buffer, the cells were incubated at room temperature for 1 h in the dark with fluorescein isothiocyanate (FITC)-labeled monoclonal anti-PC antibody (MFC-5 which recognizes the heavy chain of PC [13], 33 nM final concentration). After washing three times with the same buffer, cell-bound PC or APC was analyzed using a flow cytometer, FACScan (Becton Dickinson), and PC/APC binding as measured by the fluorescence-1 channel [21].

Amplification of DNA Fragments by Polymerase Chain Reaction (PCR)

Seven pairs of oligonucleotide PCR primers were prepared to cover all nine exons and intron–exon boundaries of PC, as described previously [17]. DNA was amplified essentially as described by Saiki et al. [22]. PCR products were either used as a template for single nucleotide primer extension or subcloned by blunt-end ligation into the pBluescript SK II(+) vector that has been linearized by *Sma*I digestion. Clones containing the desired inserts were selected after transformation using *E. coli* XLI-Blue. Single strand was prepared using helper phage R408, and then sequenced by the dideoxy chain termination method described by Sanger et al. [23] using a Sequenase version 2.0 sequencing kit and [α-^{32}P]deoxycytidine triphosphate.

Single Nucleotide Primer Extension (SNuPE)

Each SNuPE was carried out essentially as described by Kuppuswamy et al. [24]. Briefly, one cycle of PCR consisting of denaturation at 94°C for 1 min, annealing period at 60°C for 1 min, and extension at 72°C for 2 min was performed in a 25-µl reaction mixture containing about 20 ng of the amplified DNA fragment, 1 µM of the SNuPE primer, 0.5 unit of *Taq* polymerase, and 0.1 µl of the appropriate [α-^{32}P]-labeled nucleotide. The extension of the primer for each reaction was then analyzed by gel electrophoresis and autoradiography. A 6-µl aliquot of each sample was mixed with 4 µl of gel loading buffer (95% formamide, 20 mM ethylenediaminetetraacetate, 0.05% bromophenol blue, 0.05% xylene cyanol FF), heat-denatured at 90°C for 2 min, and loaded onto a 9% polyacrylamide gel containing 5.4 M urea. Electrophoresis was run at 200 V for 2 h to obtain adequate resolution of the extended primer, then the gel was dried and subjected to autoradiography.

Xba I Restriction Fragment Length Polymorphism (RFLP)

To detect the point mutation in exon III of PC gene, DNA fragments including the mutation site in exon III were amplified with a mutagenic primer, where a nucleotide T was introduced instead of G to have a new *Xba*I site in the mutant allele (T/CTAGA). PCR fragments were digested with *Xba*I and analyzed by electrophoresis (7.5% polyacrylamide gel).

Results

Antigenic and Functional Characteristics of the Patient's Protein C

The antigenic and functional levels of PC in the patient with purpura fulminans and members of his family were measured (Table 1). The total PC antigen level in the patient was 20%; however, total PC antigen level measured by ELISA using a monoclonal antibody that recognizes only the normal Gla-domain (Gla-PC antigen) was 3.8%. Amidolytic and anticoagulant activities of PC were 12.5% and less than 5%, respectively. The protein S antigen level was 83%. As shown in Table 1, the father (II-I), paternal uncle (II-2), and paternal grandmother (I-2) showed normal levels of PC antigen and normal amidolytic function, but decreased anticoagulant functions, suggesting that they have heterozygous type II PC deficiency. Furthermore, the discrepancy between the total PC antigen and

TABLE 1. Antigen and functional levels of plasma protein C in the patient's family members

| Subject | Total PC Ag | Gla-PC Ag | PC function | | PC_{clot}/PC_{amido} |
			Amidolytic	Clotting	
Normal range	70%–130%	70%–130%	80%–125%	70%–140%	
Pt (III-1)	20	3.8	12.5	<5	<0.4
II-1	97	57	84	52	0.62
II-2	70	43	62	35	0.56
I-1	97	88	93	88	0.95
I-2	117	57	81	45	0.56
II-3	48	45	43	38	0.88
II-4	117	98	101	103	1.02
I-3	90	88	78	84	1.08
I-4	57	67	63	66	1.05

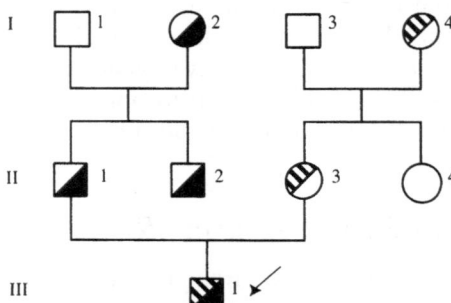

FIG. 2. Pedigree of a patient with abnormal protein C. The patient is indicated by an *arrow*. *Squares* represent male subjects, and *circles* represent female subjects. *Half-hatched* (type II protein C deficiency) and/or *half-solid* (type I protein C deficiency) symbols denote subjects heterozygous for each of two different protein C deficiencies. (From [17], with permission)

the Gla-PC antigen suggests that they have mutations in the Gla-domain. The mother (II-3) and the maternal grandmother (I-4) showed decreased PC antigen levels, as determined by two different immunoassays, and decreased PC function as determined by amidolytic and clotting assays, suggesting that they are heterozygous for the type I PC deficiency. Based on these data, the proband (III-1) may be the compound heterozygote of the two different types of abnormalities. Figure 2 shows the pedigree of the proband's family members.

Mutation Sites in Protein C Gene of the Patients

Plasmid Bluescript SK II(+) clones containing each the nine exons of the PC gene prepared from the patient were sequenced. There were two mutation sites (Fig. 3): one was a deletion of a single nucleotide G in the four consecutive G encoding Trp[380](TGG)-Gly[381](GGT) in exon IX; this abnormality would produce a frameshift mutation with complete alteration in the amino acid sequence subsequent to Val[381] in the catalytic domain of the heavy chain. This mutation was the same as that previously reported as protein C-Nagoya [25]. The other mutation was a transition from G to A in the first nucleotide of codon GAG coding for Glu[26], identified in exon III. This transition would result in a substitution of Lys

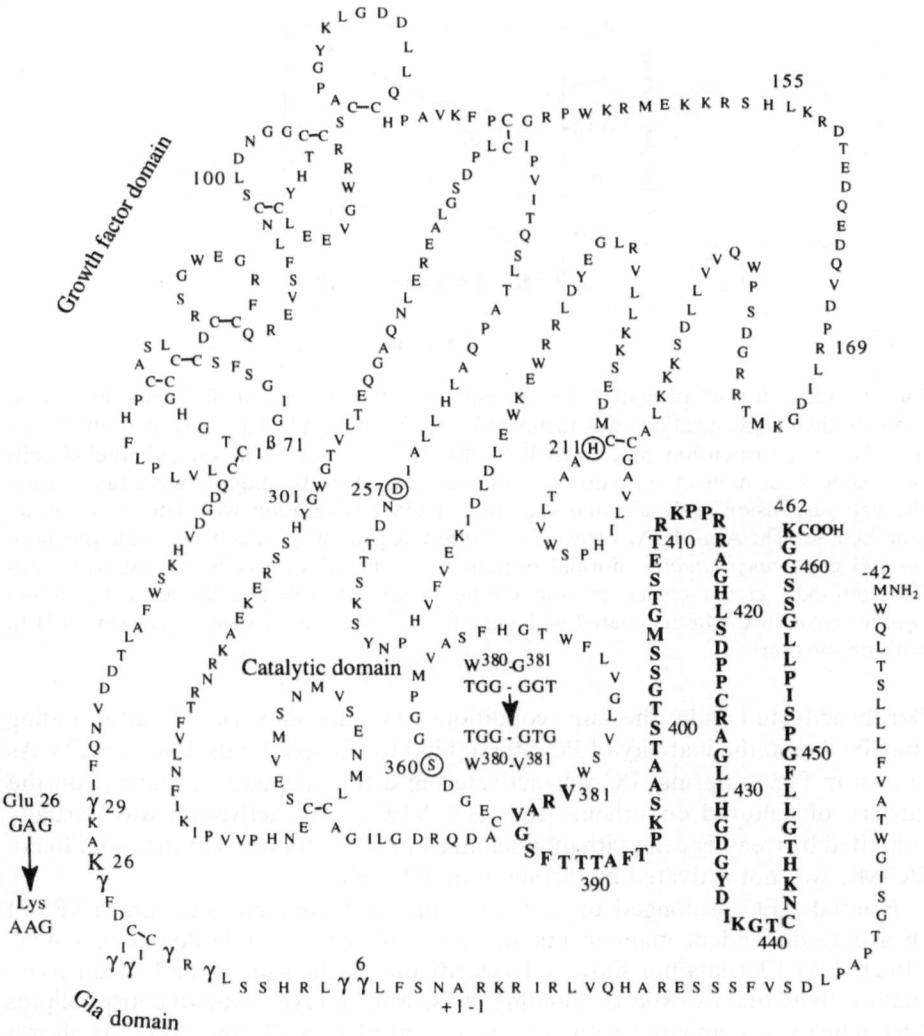

FIG. 3. Deduced amino acid sequence of abnormal protein C observed in the proband having compound heterozygous protein C deficiency

for Gla[26] in the amino acid sequence of the Gla-domain of the light chain. We termed this type of PC mutation PC-Mie.

Functional Characteristics of Protein C-Mie

The molecular basis of the functional defect of PC-Mie and APC-Mie was examined by comparing their functional characteristics with normal PC and APC. The thrombin-catalyzed activation of normal PC increased in the presence of TM, recombinant soluble TM (rsTM), and phospholipids; however, PC-Mie was

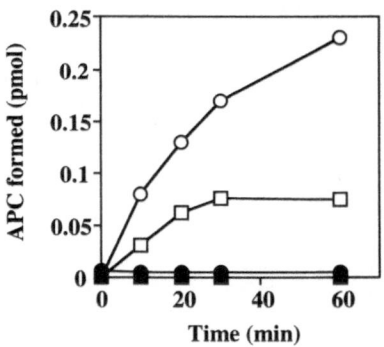

FIG. 4. Activation of protein C by thrombin on human endothelial cells. Protein C (156 nM final concentration) was incubated with thrombin (11.4 nM final concentration) at 37°C in a suspension of endothelial cells (5.5 × 10⁵ cells) or on endothelial cells pretreated with monoclonal anti-TM antibody. At intervals, aliquots were taken from the cell suspension and activated protein C (*APC*) generation was determined using Boc-Leu-Ser-Thr-Arg-MCA. *Open circles*, normal protein C incubated with the non-treated cells; *open squares*, normal protein C incubated with cells treated with anti-TM antibody; *closed circles*, protein C-Mie incubated with non-treated cells; *closed squares*, protein C-Mie incubated with cells treated with anti-TM antibody. (From [18], with permission)

hardly activated under the same conditions (data not shown). This latter finding may be due to the inability of PC-Mie to bind to phospholipids, TM, or rsTM. As shown in Fig. 4, normal PC was activated in a time-dependent manner on the surface of cultured endothelial cells (HUVECs); this activation was partially inhibited by treating cells with monoclonal anti-TM antibody. On the other hand, PC-Mie was not activated by thrombin on HUVECs.

Normal APC prolonged the activated partial thromboplastin time (APTT) in a dose-dependent manner, but neither APC-Mie nor Gla-domainless APC affected APTT (data not shown). To clarify the mechanism of the low anticoagulant activity of APC-Mie, the binding of PC-Mie and APC-Mie to phospholipids (cephalin) was compared with that of normal plasma PC and APC. As shown in Fig. 5a,b normal PC and APC bound to phospholipids fixed on microwells with apparent dissociation constants (K_ds) of 100 nM and 12 nM, respectively. However, PC-Mie and APC-Mie apparently did not bind to phospholipids. Normal APC inactivated factor Va in the presence of phospholipids, but neither APC-Mie nor Gla-domainless APC inactivated factor Va (Fig. 6). In the absence of phospholipids, factor Va was only slightly inactivated by APC.

Concerning the APC binding to protein S, APC-Mie and normal APC bound to microwell-fixed protein S with K_d values of 11.8 and 12.2 nM, respectively. In solution phase, DIP-APC-Mie and normal DIP-APC bound almost equally to biotinyl-factor Va.

The inhibition of APC-Mie and normal APC by PCI were also compared by determining the complex formation between APC and PCI using an enzyme

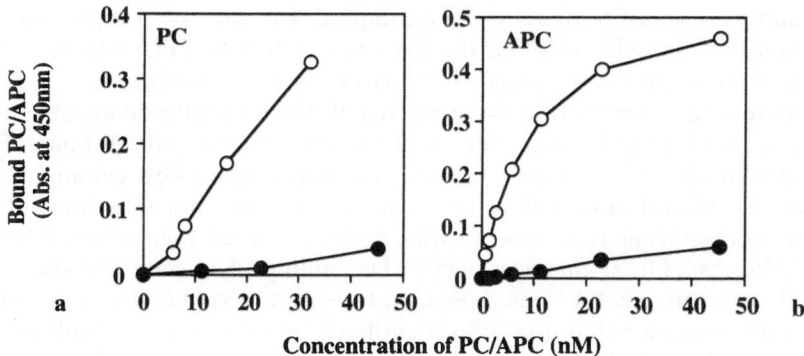

FIG. 5a,b. Binding of protein C (*PC*) and activated protein C (*APC*) to phospholipids. **a** Various concentrations of normal protein C and protein C-Mie (100 µl) were added to phospholipid-coated microwells. After washing the wells, peroxidase-coupled anti-PC F(ab)₂ was added and the peroxidase activity of the antibody bound to protein C was determined. *Open circles*, normal protein C; *closed circles*, protein C-Mie. **b** Various concentrations of normal activated protein C and activated protein C-Mie (100 µl) were added to phospholipid-coated microwells. After washing the wells, the amidolytic activity of activated protein C bound to phospholipids was determined using S-2366. *Open circles*, normal activated protein C; *closed circles*, activated protein C-Mie. (From [18], with permission)

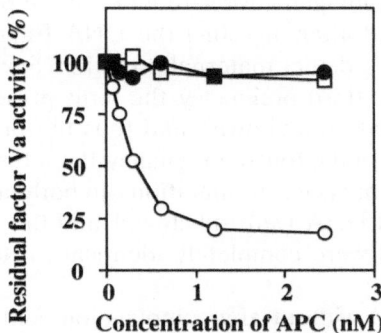

FIG. 6.   Inactivation of factor Va by normal activated protein C (*APC*) or activated protein C-Mie. Factor Va (5.5 nM) was incubated with various concentrations of normal activated protein C, Gla-domainless activated protein C, or activated protein C-Mie in 50 µl of Tris-buffered saline containing 2 mM CaCl₂ and 0.1% BSA at 37°C for 20 min. After this, 50 µl of factor V-deficient plasma was added to the mixture, then 100 µl of PT reagent was added, and clotting time was measured. *Open circles*, normal activated protein C; *open squares*, Gla-domainless activated protein C; *closed circles*, activated protein C-Mie. (From [18], with permission)

immunoassay specific for APC–PCI complex. The rate of complex formation between PCI and APC-Mie was the same as that between PCI and normal APC either in the presence or absence of heparin (data not shown).

To determine whether PC-Mie or normal PC binds to cultured human endothelial cells, each type of PC was added to the cell suspension and cell-bound PC was determined with FITC-labeled anti-PC antibody using a flow cytometer. While normal PC bound to endothelial cells, neither PC-Mie nor Gla-domainless PC bound to these cells (data not shown). A similar result was obtained for APC, APC-Mie, and Gla-domainless APC. The binding of normal PC and APC to endothelial cells was Ca^{2+}-dependent, and it was not blocked by pretreating the cells with monoclonal anti-protein S antibody or with anti-TM antibody. These binding modalities of PC and APC are in accord with those previously reported [21].

Prenatal Diagnosis of Protein C Deficiency

The proband died at 3 years old. Thereafter, the parents insisted on having a healthy baby. The second pregnancy resulted in spontaneous abortion. During the third and fourth pregnancies, we performed prenatal screening for PC abnormalities. Chorionic villi sampling and amniocentesis were done at the 10th and 17th week of gestation, respectively, and genomic DNA was isolated. To detect paternal mutation in exon III of the PC gene, we amplified DNA fragments with PCR using mutagenic forward and reverse primers. Gene analysis was performed by RFLP after digesting the DNA fragments with XbaI as described previously [17]. To detect maternal mutation, SNuPE was performed as described [17, 24]. In the third pregnancy, the fetus presented both paternal and maternal mutations (data not shown), and thus the pregnancy was terminated by artificial abortion. In the fourth pregnancy, the fetus was free from both paternal (Fig. 7a) and maternal (Fig. 7b) mutations. In both pregnancies, the PCR products derived from fetal DNA were subcloned, and the DNA sequence was determined. Data obtained were completely identical to those obtained using RFLP and SNuPE.

The pregnancy continued without any complication, and the woman underwent a cesarean section. Immediately after birth, the plasma level of Gla-PC antigen in the cord of the female baby was found to be within the normal range (data not shown). Results of the postnatal gene analysis of her PC were identical to those of the prenatal analysis.

Discussion

Hereditary deficiency of coagulant or anticoagulant factors can be caused by abnormal synthesis or by the synthesis of functionally abnormal factors. Functional abnormality of proteins provides an opportunity to examine their structure–function relationship. In the present study, we examined abnormalities of PC gene observed in a patient and in members of his family. The first mutation

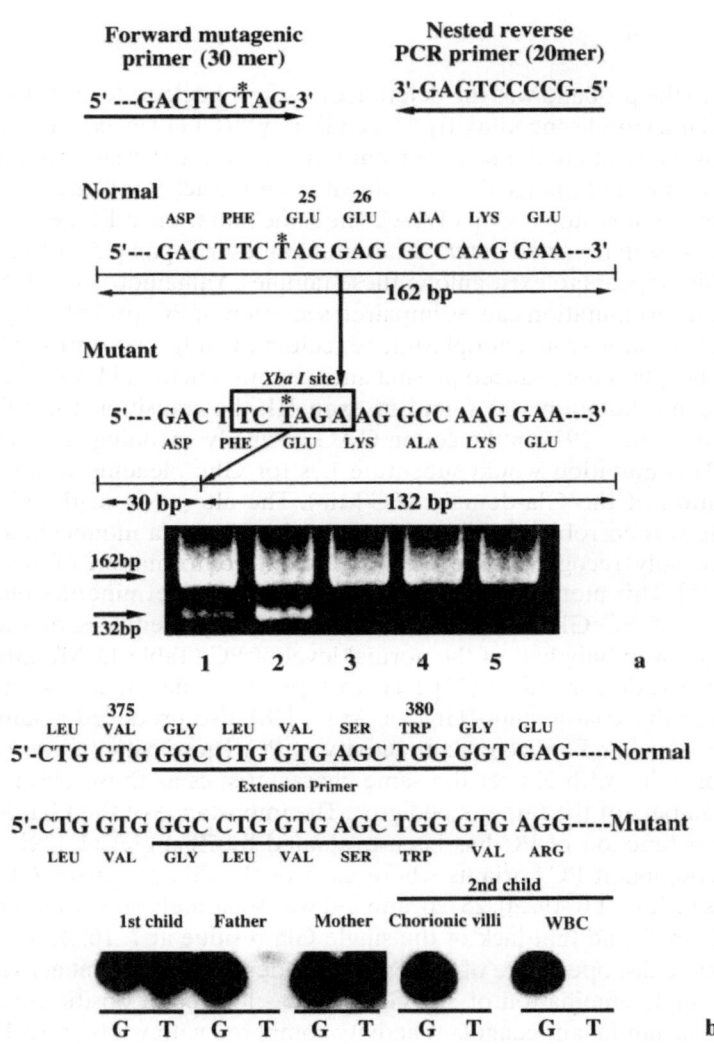

Forward mutagenic primer (30 mer)

5' ---GACTTCTAG-3'

Nested reverse PCR primer (20mer)

3'-GAGTCCCCG--5'

Normal

	25	26			
ASP	PHE	GLU	GLU	ALA	LYS	GLU

5'--- GAC T TC TAG GAG GCC AAG GAA---3'

|←——————————162 bp——————————→|

Mutant

Xba I site

5'--- GAC T TC TAG A AG GCC AAG GAA---3'

| ASP | PHE | GLU | LYS | ALA | LYS | GLU |

|←30 bp→|←——————132 bp——————→|

162bp →
132bp →

1   2   3   4   5   a

	375					380		
LEU	VAL	GLY	LEU	VAL	SER	TRP	GLY	GLU

5'-CTG GTG GGC CTG GTG AGC TGG GGT GAG-----Normal

Extension Primer

5'-CTG GTG GGC CTG GTG AGC TGG GTG AGG-----Mutant

| LEU | VAL | GLY | LEU | VAL | SER | TRP | VAL | ARG |

2nd child

1st child   Father   Mother   Chorionic villi   WBC

G T   G T   G T   G T   G T   b

Fig. 7a,b. Prenatal diagnosis of protein C deficiency. **a** Detection of point mutation in exon III of protein C gene by restriction fragment length polymorphism. DNA fragments including whole exon III were amplified and used as a template in the second polymerase chain reaction (PCR). To create a new *Xba*I site in the mutant allele, G was replaced by T (indicated by *asterisks*) (mutagenic primer). By using forward mutagenic primer and reverse nested primer, DNA fragments were amplified, digested with *Xba*I, and electrophoresed on 7.5% polyacrylamide gel. The digested fragment (132 bp) was detected in the mutant allele, whereas the normal allele was uncut (162 bp). Lanes: *1*, the proband; *2*, father; *3*, mother; *4*, chorionic villi of the fourth pregnancy; *5*, peripheral blood of the baby. **b** The deletion of one G in the four consecutive G of exon IX was detected by single nucleotide primer extension. DNA fragments in exon IX were amplified from genomic DNA and used as a template for single nucleotide primer extension. One cycle of PCR was performed using the primer (*underline*) and either [32P] deoxyguanosine triphosphate (to detect normal allele) or [32P] thymidine triphosphate (to detect mutant allele), and analyzed using 9% polyacrylamide gel containing 5.4 M urea (From [30], with permission)

observed in the proband was the deletion of a single nucleotide G in the four consecutive G nucleotide encoding Trp[380](TGG)–Gly[381](GGT) in exon IX of PC gene.
This abnormality alters the residue from Gly[381] to Val and results in a frameshift
mutation that would change the subsequent 39 amino acids and add 42 new amino
acids up to the next stop codon (TAA). The same mutation in PC gene, called PC-
Nagoya, has been reported in two different families in Japan [25, 26], although no
relationship appears to exist among these families. Yamamoto et al. [25] demonstrated that this mutation causes impaired secretion of PC, probably by obstructing its translocation from endoplasmic reticulum to Golgi apparatus in liver cells;
this would explain the reduced plasma antigen and functional level of PC.

The second mutation was found in exon III: the transition from G to A at
nucleotide number 2977 in the codon GAG normally encoding Glu[26] in the Gla-
domain. This mutation would substitute Lys for Glu[26], leading to an abnormal
conformation of the Gla-domain (PC-Mie). The alteration in the Gla-domain
of PC-Mie was corroborated by its defective binding to a monoclonal antibody
that specifically recognizes the Ca^{2+}-dependent conformation of the PC Gla-
domain [15]. This monoclonal antibody was used to determine the plasma concentrations of PC Gla-domain. The affected family members of the father's
pedigree showed only half of the normal level of PC (Table 1). Mutations in the
Gla-domain (Ala for Gla[20]) [27] lead to type II PC deficiency. Another point
mutation in the Gla-domain (Gly for Arg[15]) [28] also produced a similar effect
on antigen level and anticoagulant activity of PC. These patients present abnormal PC proteins with almost the same characteristics as those observed in the
family members of the father's pedigree. The importance of the Gla-domain for
the normal function of PC has been evaluated by Zhang et al. [29]. They prepared recombinant PC variants where each of the Gla precursor Glu residues
(positions 6, 7, 14, I 6, 19, 20, 25, 26, and 29) was separately substituted by an Asp
residue. They found that lack of the single Gla residue at 7, 16, 20, or 26 results
in a complete disappearance of the Ca^{2+}-dependent anticoagulant activity. On the
contrary, single elimination of any Gla residues located at positions 6, 14, or 19
retained substantial anticoagulant activity compared with wild-type APC. Therefore, it is likely that Glu residues at positions 7, 16, 20, and 26 are essential for
maintaining the conformation of Gla-domain.

The observation that PC-Mie has impaired anticoagulant activity is probably
not surprising in view of the several properties that PC-Mie shares with Gla-
domainless PC. First, the Gla-domain is responsible for the PC binding to phospholipids; the PC-Mie essentially does not bind to phospholipids. Second, in the
presence of phospholipids, purified factor Va is inactivated by normal APC but
not by APC-Mie or Gla-domainless APC. In the absence of phospholipids, factor
Va is only slightly inactivated by APC. Furthermore, recombinant Gla-domain
PC mutants, including a mutant having substitution of Asp for Glu[26], showed
decreased binding to phospholipids. Therefore, Gla[26] of PC is essential for binding
to phospholipids. It is possible that APC-Mie does not bind to protein S, which
may result in defective inactivation of factor Va by APC-Mie. This appears
unlikely for two reasons: first, APC-Mie and normal APC bind equally to protein

S fixed to microwells. Second, there was a significant difference in the inactivation capacity of factor Va between APC-Mie and normal APC even in the absence of protein S. Thus, this missense mutation would alter the conformation of the Gla-domain and result in a reduced anticoagulant but normal amidolytic activities.

Since the Gla-domain of PC plays an important role in PC activation, it is conceivable that the Gla-domain directly interacts with TM. A possible role for the PC Gla-domain in the activation process is suggested by several findings described here. First, in the presence of Ca^{2+}, normal PC directly interacts with TM or rsTM which lacks a binding site for phospholipid. Second, PC-Mie, which has a defective Gla-domain, does not bind to TM. Third, addition of purified Gla-domain in the reaction mixture resulted in a dose-dependent inhibition of thrombin-catalyzed PC activation in the presence of rsTM alone, and in the presence of TM and phospholipid. Taken together, these findings suggest the occurrence of a direct interaction between the Gla-domain of PC and TM.

Recently, PC receptor has been identified on endothelial cell membrane [21]. The structural and functional importance of the Gla-domain of PC is extended by the present study showing that PC not only interacts with phospholipids, but also with TM or PC receptor. PC-Mie failed to interact with PC receptor. The Gla-domainless PC had a similar effect on PC receptor binding. Therefore, it is likely that PC directly interacts with PC receptor, the Ca^{2+}-dependent Gla-domain probably playing a major role in this interaction.

The two PC mutations described in the present study must be functionally important because the patient developed severe neonatal purpura fulminans. The only way to avoid giving birth to a neonate with this disease as a consequence of severe PC deficiency is by prenatal diagnosis. In this study we could diagnose abnormalities in PC gene using PCR with subsequent RFLP or SNuPE. These diagnostic methods are accurate and rapid.

Acknowledgment. We thank Dr. Esteban C. Gabazza for his helpful comments on the manuscript.

References

1. Stenflo J (1976) A new vitamin K-dependent protein. Purification from bovine plasma and preliminary characterization. J Biol Chem 251:355–363
2. Kisiel W (1979) Human plasma protein C: isolation, characterization, and mechanism of activation by alpha-thrombin. J Clin Invest 64:761–769
3. Esmon NL, Owen WG, Esmon CT (1982) Isolation of a membrane-bound cofactor for thrombin-catalyzed activation of protein C. J Biol Chem 257:859–864
4. Esmon CT (1987) The regulation of natural anticoagulant pathways. Science 235:1348–1352
5. Esmon CT (1989) The roles of protein C and thrombomodulin in the regulation of blood coagulation. J Biol Chem 264:4743–4746

6. de Foun N, Haverkate F, Bertina RM, Koopman J, van Wijngddrden A, van Hinsbergh
   V (1986) The cofactor role of protein S in the acceleration of whole blood clot lysis
   by activated protein C in vitro. Blood 67:1189–1192
7. Suzuki K, Stenflo J, Dahlback B, Teodorsson B (1983) Inactivation of human coagulation factor V by activated protein C. J Biol Chem 258:1914–1920
8. van Hinsbergh V, Bertina RM, van Wijngddrden A, van Tilburg N, Emeis JJ,
   Haverkate F (1985) Activated protein C decreases plasminogen activator-inhibitor
   activity in endothelial cellconditioned medium. Blood 65:444–451
9. Bajzar L, Nesheim M, Morser J, Tracy PB (1998) Both cellular and soluble forms
   of thrombomodulin inhibit fibrinolysis by potentiating the activation of thrombin-
   activable fibrinolysis inhibitor. J Biol Chem 273:2792–2798
10. Plutzky J, Hoskins JA, Long GL, Crabtree GR (1986) Evolution and organization
    of the human protein C gene. Proc Natl Acad Sci USA 83:546–550
11. Broekmans AW, Veltkamp JJ, Bertina RM (1983) Congenital protein C deficiency
    and venous thromboembolism. A study of three Dutch families. N Engl J Med
    309:340–344
12. Marlar RA, Mastovich S (1990) Hereditary protein C deficiency: a review of the
    genetics, clinical presentation, diagnosis and treatment. Blood Coagul Fibrinolysis
    1:319–330
13. Suzuki K, Matsuda Y, Kusumoto H, Nishioka J, Terada M, Yamashita T, Hashimoto S
    (1985) Monoclonal antibodies to human protein C: effects on the biological activity
    of activated protein C and the thrombin-catalyzed activation of protein C1. J Biochem
    (Tokyo) 97:127–138
14. Suzuki K, Hayashi T, Koyama M, Yoshimura T, Shimamoto M, Kimura N, Kita M
    (1989) Rapid homogeneous enzyme immunoassay of plasma protein C. Clin Chim
    Acta 184:227–233
15. Wakabayashi K, Sakata Y, Aoki N (1986) Conformation-specific monoclonal anti-
    bodies to the calcium-induced structure of protein C. J Biol Chem 261:11 097–11 105
16. Martinoli JL, Stocker K (1986) Fast functional protein C assay using Protac, a novel
    protein C activator. Thromb Res 43:253–264
17. Ido M, Ohiwa M, Hayashi T, Nishioka J, Hatada T, Watanabe Y, Wada H, Shirakawa
    S, Suzuki K (1993) A compound heterozygous protein C deficiency with a single
    nucleotide G deletion encoding Gly-381 and an amino acid substitution of Lys for
    Gla-26. Thromb Haemost 70:636–641
18. Nishioka J, Ido M, Hayashi T, Suzuki K (1996) The Gla26 residue of protein C is
    required for the binding of protein C to thrombomodulin and endothelial cell protein
    C receptor, but not to protein S and factor Va. Thromb Haemost 75:275–282
19. Suzuki K, Hayashi T, Nishioka J, Kosaka Y, Zushi M, Honda G, Yamamoto S (1989)
    A domain composed of epidermal growth factor-like structures of human thrombo-
    modulin is essential for thrombin binding and for protein C activation. J Biol Chem
    264:4872–4876
20. Suzuki K, Nishioka J, Hashimoto S (1983) Protein C inhibitor. Purification from
    human plasma and characterization. J Biol Chem 258:163–168
21. Fukudome K, Esmon CT (1994) Identification, cloning, and regulation of a novel
    endothelial cell protein C/activated protein C receptor. J Biol Chem 269:26486–
    26491
22. Saiki RK, Gelfand DH, Stoffel S, Scharf SJ, Higuchi R, Horn GT, Mullis KB, Erlich
    HA (1988) Primer-directed enzymatic amplification of DNA with a thermostable
    DNA polymerase. Science 239:487–491

23. Sanger F, Nicklen S, Coulson AR (1977) DNA sequencing with chain-terminating inhibitors. Proc Natl Acad Sci USA 74:5463–5467
24. Kuppuswamy MN, Hoffmann JW, Kasper CK, Spitzer SG, Groce SL, Bajaj SP (1991) Single nucleotide primer extension to detect genetic diseases: experimental application to hemophilia B (factor IX) and cystic fibrosis genes. Proc Natl Acad Sci USA 88:1143–1147
25. Yamamoto K, Tanimoto M, Emi N, Matsushita T, Takamatsu J, Saito H (1992) Impaired secretion of the elongated mutant of protein C (protein C-Nagoya). Molecular and cellular basis for hereditary protein C deficiency. J Clin Invest 90:2439–2446
26. Tokunaga F, Wakabayashi S, Sato H, Arakawa M, Tawaraya H, Koide T (1992) Identification of one base deletion in exon IX of the protein C gene that causes a type I deficiency. Thromb Res 68:417–423
27. Bovill EG, Tomczak JA, Grant B, Bhushan F, Pillemer E, Rainville IR, Long GL (1992) Protein CVermont: symptomatic type II protein C deficiency associated with two GLA domain mutations. Blood 79:1456–1465
28. Mimuro J, Muramatsu S, Kaneko M, Yoshitake S, Iijima K, Nakamura K, Sakata Y, Matsuda M (1993) An abnormal protein C (protein C Yonago) with an amino acid substitution of Gly for Arg-15 caused by a single base mutation of C to G in codon 57 (CGG → GGG). Deteriorated calcium-dependent conformation of the gamma-carboxyglutamic acid domain relevant to a thrombotic tendency. Int J Hematol 57:9–14
29. Zhang L, Jhingan A, Castellino FJ (1992) Role of individual gamma-carboxyglutamic acid residues of activated human protein C in defining its in vitro anticoagulant activity. Blood 80:942–952
30. Ido M, Hayashi T, Nishioka J, Itoh M, Minoura H, Toyoda N, Hirayama M, Kawasaki H, Sakurai M, Suzuki K (1996) Prenatal diagnosis of compound heterozygous deficiency of protein C by direct detection of the mutation sites. Thromb Haemost 76:277–278

Activated Protein C Resistance, Factor V Leiden, and Venous Thromboembolism

PAUL M. RIDKER and DANIEL T. PRICE

Summary. Factor V Leiden mutation is the most common inherited defect of coagulation currently known, with a prevalence between 3% and 6% in Caucasian populations. The result of a single adenine-for-guanine point mutation in the gene coding for coagulation factor V, factor V Leiden leads to a hypercoagulable state in part by rendering a key binding site on coagulation factor Va partially resistant to the anticoagulant effects of activated protein C. Clinically, this state is referred to as activated protein C resistance. Individuals affected by factor V Leiden appear to be at significantly increased risks of first and recurrent venous thrombosis, particularly those events not associated with cancer, surgery, or trauma. Moreover, risks of venous thrombosis among carriers of factor V Leiden dramatically increase in the presence of other acquired coagulation defects including hyperhomocysteinemia and oral contraceptive use. Screening programs for factor V Leiden must carefully consider the prevalence of mutation in a given population, the absolute as well as relative risks imparted by the mutation, and the benefit-to-risk ratio associated with any therapeutic intervention based upon a positive test finding. Ongoing clinical studies such as the Prevention of Recurrent Venous Thromboembolism (PREVENT) trial will help to determine whether individuals who carry factor V Leiden and have had a first venous thrombosis should be considered for chronic, low-dose anticoagulation therapy.

Keywords. Thrombosis, Factor V Leiden, Activated protein C resistance, Coagulation, Hypercoagulability

Introduction

Until recently, genetic risk factors for venous thromboembolism were rarely considered in the standard clinical evaluation of patients suffering deep vein thrombosis and pulmonary embolism. Rather, patients suspected of harboring a

Cardiovascular Division, Brigham and Women's Hospital, Harvard Medical School (PMR), and the Section of Cardiology, Boston University Medical Center (DTP), Boston, MA 02115, USA

hypercoagulable state were traditionally evaluated for plasma-based defects associated with protein S or protein C deficiencies, disorders of antithrombin III, dysfibrinogenemias, and acquired abnormalities including hyperhomocysteinemia, antiphospholipid antibodies, and the lupus anticoagulant [1] (Table 1). However, with the discovery in 1993 of a common inherited disorder associated with activated protein C resistance [2–4], interest in inherited causes of thrombophilia greatly increased. Indeed, the recognition that as many as half of all cases of familial thrombosis are associated with activated protein C resistance rapidly led to the discovery that this defect is usually the result of a single base pair mutation in the factor V gene commonly referred to as factor V Leiden [5–7].

Recent studies in unselected patient groups indicate that factor V Leiden is common among Caucasians, with a prevalence between 3% and 6% [8], but is much less frequent among Asian and African populations [8–11]. Clinically, factor V Leiden is associated with significantly increased risks of first [12] as well as

TABLE 1. Primary and secondary causes of venous thrombosis

A. Primary hypercoagulable states
    Antithrombin disorders
        Antithrombin deficiency
    Protein C/ protein S disorders
        Protein C deficiency
        Protein S deficiency
        Resistance to activated protein C
    Fibrinolytic disorders
        Hypoplasminogenemia
        Dyplasminogenemia
        Disorders of plasminogen activation (tPA/PAI-1)
        Dysfibrinogenemia
    Common genetic disorders of hemostasis
        Factor V Leiden
        Prothrombin mutation

B. Secondary hypercoagulable states
    Abnormalities of blood flow
        Venous stasis
        Obesity
        Surgery
        Trauma
    Abnormalities of vessel wall function
        Hyperhomocysteinemia
        Antiphospholipid syndromes
    Abnormalities of coagulation
        Pregnancy
        Oral contraceptive use
        Nephrotic syndrome
        Myeloproliferative disorders / cancer

Adapted from [1].

recurrent [13, 14] venous thromboses. However, whether physicians should screen for factor V Leiden remains controversial, and it is currently uncertain whether factor V Leiden carriers should be considered for more intense or more prolonged periods of anticoagulation following events of venous thromboembolism.

In this chapter, an overview of activated protein C resistance and factor V Leiden is provided which emphasizes the clinical implications of these recently described determinants of hypercoagulability [15]. In addition, the rationale for considering long-term versus short-term anticoagulation in the secondary prevention of venous thromboses among those who carry factor V Leiden is presented [16].

Activated Protein C Resistance and Factor V Leiden

When activated, coagulation factor V (factor Va) is a potent procoagulant protein which leads to an amplification of the coagulation pathway, ultimately resulting in the formation of fibrin. In most individuals, the activity of factor Va is modulated by the naturally occurring anticoagulant, activated protein C. However, in some patients, binding of activated protein C to factor Va is partially reduced, leading to a clinical state known as activated protein C resistance [2–4]. This reduced binding is almost always due to a single adenine for guanine point mutation in the gene coding for coagulation factor V which leads to arginine being replaced by glutamine at nucleotide position 506 [5–7]. This site is one of the three cleavage sites on factor V for activated protein C. Commonly known as the factor V Leiden mutation, this genetic defect results in a form of factor Va that is relatively resistant to degradation by activated protein C, leading to a hypercoagulable state [17] (Fig. 1).

Testing for the laboratory abnormality of activated protein C resistance is relatively simple and can be performed by measurement of the activated partial thromboplastin time (aPTT) in the presence and absence of activated protein C [18]. In general, results of these assays are presented as a ratio with low levels (<2.0) being associated with an increased predisposition to thrombosis. Initially, assays for activated protein C resistance were of limited value among patients on warfarin or heparin or among those known to carry the lupus anticoagulant. However, clinical assays are now widely available which employ factor V-deficient plasma and allow for assessment of activated protein C resistance in most patient groups [19–22].

A reduced activated protein C resistance ratio correlates well with heterozygosity or homozygosity for the factor V Leiden mutation (Fig. 2). In most clinical settings, a definitive genetic diagnosis of factor V Leiden mutation status is made with polymerase chain reaction-based techniques [5–7]. Since some forms of activated protein C resistance appear to be acquired, genetic confirmation for the presence or absence of factor V Leiden mutation is often recommended for

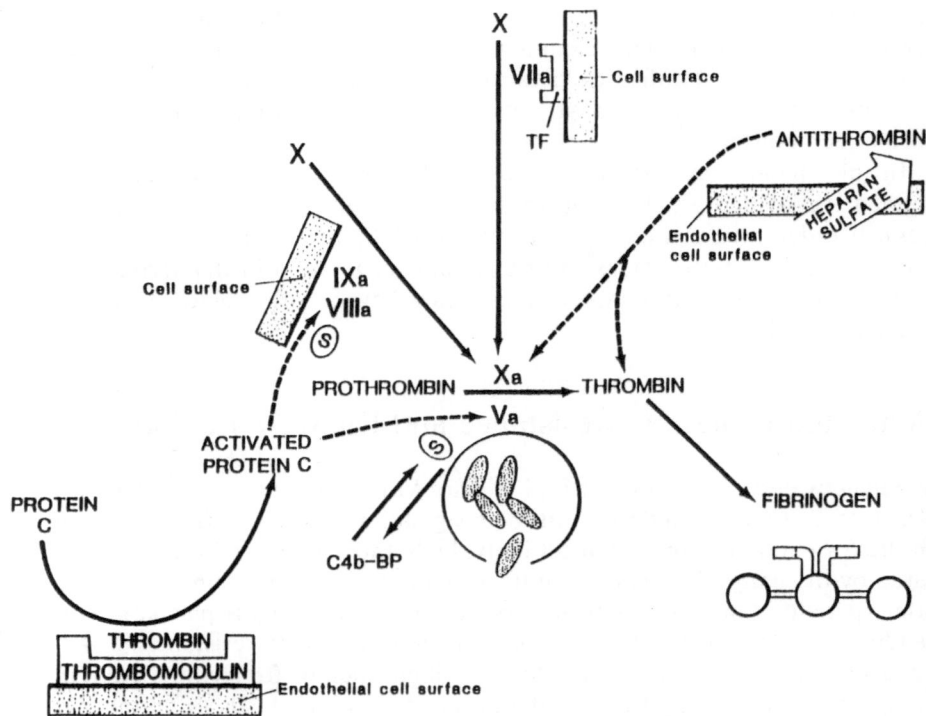

FIG. 1. Pathways that generate factor Xa and thrombin and the natural anticoagulant mechanisms that regulate activity of these enzymes. Note the critical role of activated protein C as a naturally occurring anticoagulant which normally inactivates factors VIIIa and Va. Factor V Leiden mutation results in a form of coagulation factor V that, when activated to factor Va, is relatively resistant to degradation by activated protein C. (From [63], with permission)

those with a positive plasma-based test for activated protein C resistance and a history of venous thrombosis [15]. Genetic studies are also of value in determining risks for family members of affected individuals.

In the largest cross-sectional study completed to date, a group of 4047 randomly selected Americans were screened for factor V Leiden to determine the population prevalence of this common mutation [8]. Overall, the carrier frequency for the factor V Leiden mutation was 3.7% in this study (allele frequency 1.9%). However, important ethnic specific differences in gene frequency were observed such that the prevalence of factor V Leiden mutation was highest among Caucasian Americans (5.3%), and significantly less prevalent among other ethnic groups. In particular, the factor V leiden mutation was found in only 1% of African-Americans and less than 0.5% of Asian-Americans [8]. These differences may explain in part observations of lower risks of venous thrombosis among these latter patient groups [9–11, 23].

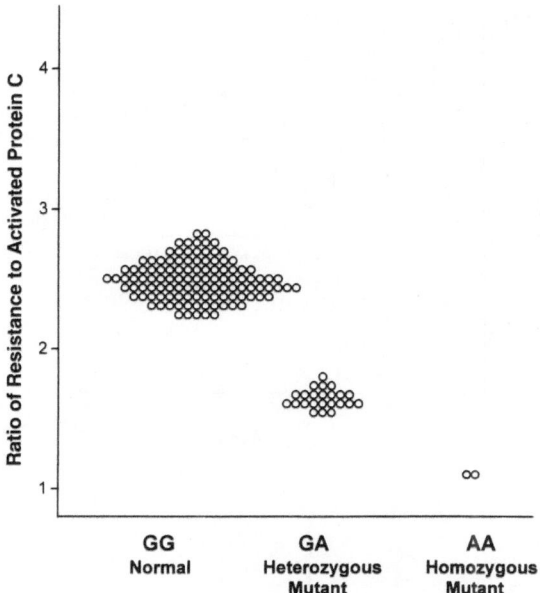

FIG. 2. The relationship between activated protein C resistance ratios and carrier states for factor V Leiden mutation. *A*, adenine; *G*, guanine. (From [15], with permission)

Factor V Leiden and Risks of Venous Thromboembolism

Clinical studies of patients with recurrent familial thrombosis led to the initial recognition of a relationship between the factor V Leiden mutation and venous thromboembolism [2, 3]. For example, in one study of patients with familial thrombosis, markedly reduced rates of thrombosis-free survival were observed among those both heterozygous and homozygous for the factor V Leiden mutation [24] (Fig. 3). In referral populations of unexplained juvenile or recurrent thrombosis, the overall prevalence of activated protein C resistance may be as high as 50% [25].

The Leiden Thrombophilia Study demonstrated convincingly that resistance to activated protein C is a risk factor for thromboembolism in the general population. In this population-based case-controlled study of patients with a first episode of nonmalignancy-associated deep vein thrombosis, there was a seven-fold increase in risk of deep vein thrombosis in those demonstrating activated protein C resistance [4]. Subsequent genetic analysis demonstrated that the majority of these activated protein C-resistant individuals were heterozygous or homozygous for the factor V Leiden mutation [5]. The high correlation between activated protein C resistance and factor V Leiden mutation has since been supported by several other studies.

The prospective Physicians Health Study provided genetic confirmation that factor V Leiden was the most common inherited defect of thrombosis known [12]. In that study of nearly 15 000 individuals free of cardiovascular disease or cancer, 121 cases of venous thromboembolism occurred over a mean follow-up

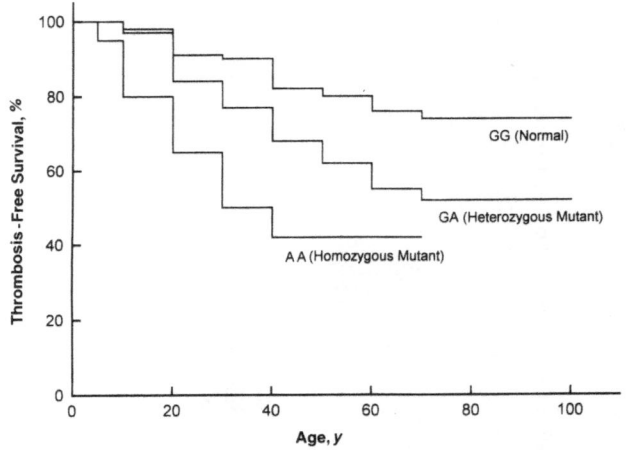

Fig. 3. Thrombosis-free survival in patients with familial thrombophilia. *A*, adenine; *G*, guanine. Adapted from [24]

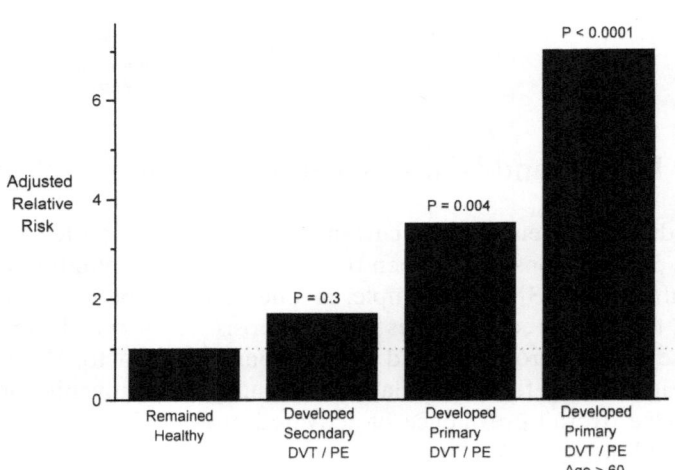

Fig. 4. Relative risks of future venous thrombosis among apparently healthy men associated with factor V Leiden mutation. Adapted from [12]. DVT/PE, deep vein thrombosis/ pulmonary embolism

period of 8.6 years. The overall relative risk of the mutation among men with venous thromboembolism was 2.7. However, in those with idiopathic events, the risk imparted by the mutation was substantially higher, particularly in the subgroup of older individuals [12] (Fig. 4). There did not appear to be an association between factor V Leiden mutation and secondary thromboembolism (i.e., those events associated with surgery, trauma, or cancer). No association was observed in this prospective study between factor V Leiden and risks of myocardial infarction or stroke.

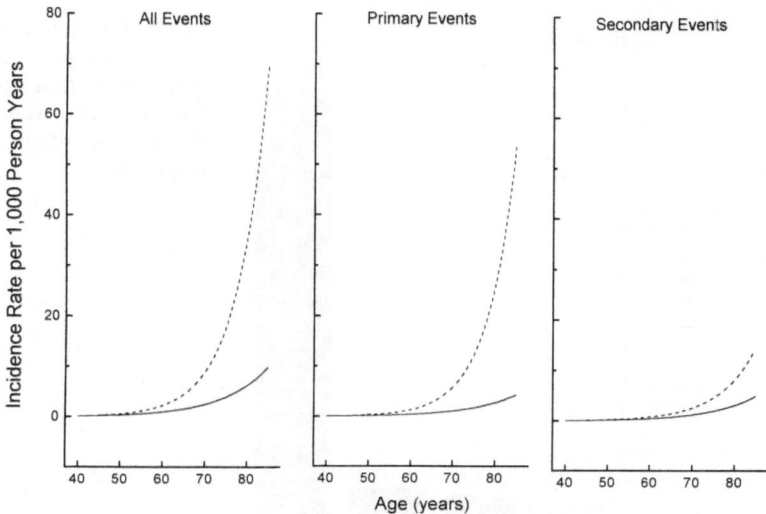

FIG. 5. Estimated age-specific incidence rates for venous thrombosis among men with (*dashed lines*) and without (*solid lines*) factor V Leiden mutation. *Left* Any venous thrombosis; *middle* idiopathic venous thrombosis; *right* venous thrombosis associated with cancer or surgery. Adapted from [27]

Those homozygous for factor V Leiden mutation, as may be expected, appear to be at even higher risk. For example, it has been estimated that the risk of venous thromboembolism among patients homozygous for factor V Leiden mutation may be increased as much as 80-fold [26]. Further, patients homozygous for factor V Leiden mutation appear to present with initial thromboembolism at a younger age than those heterozygous or unaffected by the mutation. Homozygosity for factor V Leiden, however, is a rare condition. In contrast, among patients who are heterozygous carriers of factor V Leiden, risks of venous thromboembolism appear to increase with age [27] (Fig. 5). This observation suggests that acquired abnormalities of coagulation are also important determinants of thrombosis risk and that the risks associated with such abnormalities are at least additive to that associated with factor V Leiden [15].

For example, patients with both hyperhomocystinemia and factor V Leiden appear to have risks of venous thrombosis 20 times that of individuals with neither defect such that the risks of venous thromboembolism in doubly affected persons is significantly greater than the risk associated with either condition alone [28] (Fig. 6). Similarly, women on oral contraceptives who also carry factor V Leiden have been reported to have a 30- to 35-fold increase in risk of venous thrombosis [29] (Fig. 7). However, despite these increased relative risks, the absolute risk of venous thrombosis among women on oral contraception remains low, and screening programs prior to prescription of oral contraceptives are unlikely to produce a net clinical benefit [15, 30–32]. It is currently uncertain

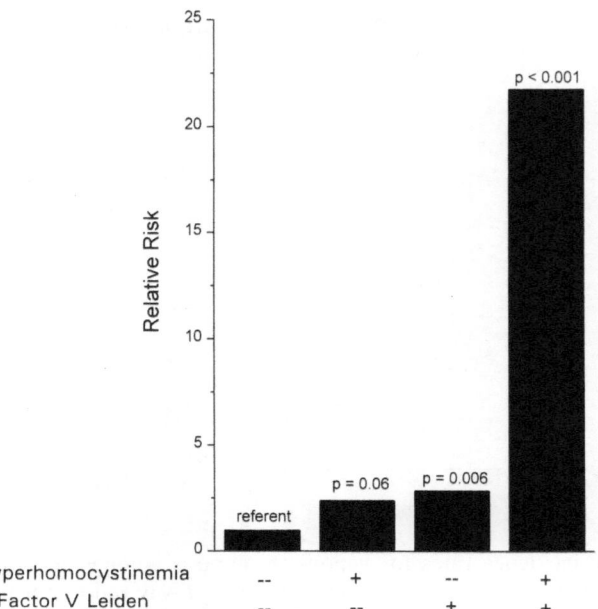

FIG. 6. Interrelation of factor V Leiden mutation and hyperhomocysteinemia on risks of venous thrombosis. Adapted from [28]

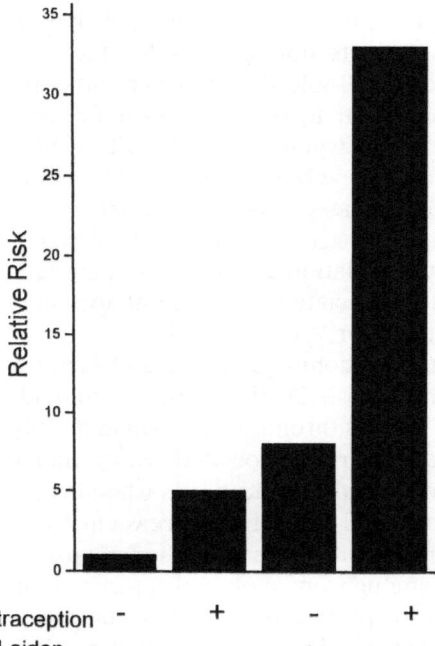

FIG. 7. Interrelation of factor V Leiden and oral contraceptive use on risks of venous thrombosis. Adapted from [29]

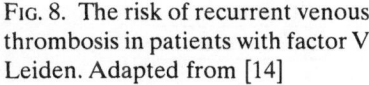

FIG. 8. The risk of recurrent venous thrombosis in patients with factor V Leiden. Adapted from [14]

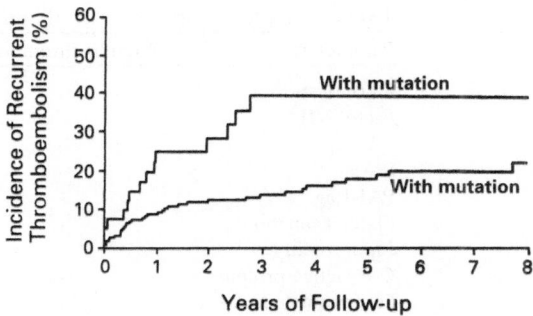

Years of Follow-up

whether factor V Leiden interacts with postmenopausal estrogen replacement therapy.

Several studies document the fact that patients with factor V Leiden who have had a first venous thrombosis are at substantially increased risks for recurrent events [13, 14]. For example, in one recent prospective study of survivors of an initial idiopathic venous thromboembolism [13], those affected by factor V Leiden mutation were four times more likely to suffer a recurrent event compared to those without the mutation. Indeed, in that study, 76% of the recurrent events were attributable to factor V Leiden mutation [13]. Similarly, in a study with long-term follow-up, those with factor V Leiden were more than twice as likely to suffer a recurrent event [14] (Fig. 8). In both of these studies, the great majority of recurrent venous thromboembolic events occurred after cessation of standard anticoagulant therapy.

Factor V Leiden and Risks of Arterial Thrombosis

In contrast to venous thrombosis, data relating activated protein C resistance and factor V Leiden to risks of arterial thrombosis have been inconsistent. For example, while several early case series suggested an association between factor V Leiden and myocardial infarction [33], most large-scale studies have not confirmed this observation [12, 34–36]. Similarly, while some data suggest an association between factor V Leiden and stroke [37, 38], most studies have again found no association [12, 39]. Small hypothesis-generating studies have suggested a potential role for factor V Leiden in arterial thrombosis among young women with concomitant risk factors such as smoking and oral contraceptive use [40]. This finding, however, has not been confirmed in large-scale studies.

The observation that factor V Leiden is a potent risk factor for venous thrombosis but appears to have a marginal role in arterial thrombosis provides an important insight into the differences between thrombosis in the arterial and venous circulations [41]. As outlined in Table 2, plasma-based risk factors asso-

TABLE 2. Risk factors for arterial and venous thrombosis

Parameter	Venous thrombosis	Arterial thrombosis
Fibrinogen	−	+++
Factor VII	−	+
vWF:ag	−	++
tPA:ag	−	+++
PAI-1:ag	−	++
Platelet function	−	++
Lipoprotein (a)	−	+
C-Reactive protein	−	+++
Serum amyloid A	−	++
APC Resistance	+++	−
Factor V Leiden	+++	−
Prothrombin mutation	++	−
Factor VIII	++	−
Antithrombin III	++	−
Protein C	++	−
Protein S	++	−
Homocysteine	++	++
D-Dimer	++	++

ciated with impaired fibrinolysis such as abnormalities of tissue-type plasminogen activator have been shown to be potent predictors of both myocardial infarction [42] and stroke [43], but appear to have little role in venous disease [44]. Similarly, inflammatory risk factors such as fibrinogen [45] and C-reactive protein [46, 47], which are strong independent predictors of arterial thrombosis, have not proven to be associated with venous disease. Thus, differences between atherosclerotic associated thrombosis in the arterial system and stasis-related hypercoagulability in the venous system appear to be two distinct pathologic processes.

Factor V Leiden and the Duration and Intensity of Anticoagulant Therapy

A critical issue in the management of patients with venous thrombosis is the duration of anticoagulant therapy required to prevent recurrent events [48]. Based on available data, current treatment recommendations from the American College of Chest Physicians includes heparinization for 5 to 7 days followed by at least 3 months of oral anticoagulation with warfarin targeting the international normalized ratio (INR) between 2.0 and 3.0 [49]. However, patients following these recommendations experience high rates of recurrent thrombosis, rehospitalization, and mortality following the cessation of anticoagulant therapy.

One clinical approach to this problem has been to increase the duration of warfarin therapy to 6 months, a strategy which has proven highly successful in reducing rates of recurrent venous thromboembolism [50] (Fig. 9). However, rates of

FIG. 9. Effects of 6 months versus 6 weeks of oral anticoagulation in the prevention of recurrent venous thrombosis. Adapted from [50]

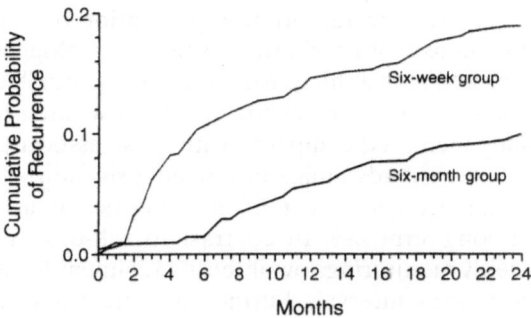

bleeding during such a prolonged period of full-dose anticoagulation are increased and the net clinical benefit of such an approach remains uncertain. Moreover, even after a 6-month period of anticoagulation, recurrent events remain a problem. For example, in one recent evaluation, almost one-quarter of all study subjects experienced a recurrent venous thromboembolic event within 2 years of drug cessation [51, 52]. Other prospective studies indicate that these risks are predominantly limited to those individuals in whom the index event was not associated with cancer, surgery, or trauma [12, 13, 52]. It has been hypothesized that risks of recurrent events are even higher among those with known inherited defects of anticoagulation. In particular, recurrence rates for those with the factor V Leiden mutation may be as high as 40% over a 3- to 4-year period [14].

While data describing the long-term risks of recurrent venous thrombosis are remarkably consistent, virtually no data are available outlining the utility of chronic anticoagulation beyond a 6-month period. Many clinicians are wary about long-term anticoagulation because of concern about ongoing risks for hemorrhage, particularly when full-dose warfarin (INR 2.0–3.0) is employed [16]. Such concerns appear justified. For example, one secondary prevention trial of venous thrombosis which employed an "indefinite treatment" arm reported a 9% rate of major or fatal hemorrhage [53]. These risks appear to increase in the elderly, a group at particularly high risk for recurrent events. In this regard, the National Consortium of Anticoagulation Clinics registry reports a 7% to 9% rate of major or fatal hemorrhage for every 100 patient-years of treatment with full-dose warfarin therapy [54]. Complication rates in these data increased directly with increasing age.

To lower these hemorrhagic risks, several investigators have considered low-intensity warfarin (INR 1.5–2.0) for secondary prevention studies [16]. Such an approach has several potential advantages. First, the safety of low-dose warfarin has been well documented. In the Coumadin Aspirin Reinfarction Study, for example, patients randomly assigned to low-intensity warfarin were found to have similar levels of hemoglobin and hematocrit when compared with those randomly assigned to placebo, and the most common adverse side effect of microscopic hematuria was not related to the INR level achieved [55, 56]. Similarly, in a recently reported primary prevention of ischemic heart disease trial [57, 58], low-intensity warfarin was given on a prolonged basis (up to 10 years) to several thousand men at high risk for first myocardial infarction. In this large-scale study, absolute risks of hemorrhage with low-intensity warfarin were small and minimally increased compared with those associated with aspirin alone [58].

A second advantage of low-intensity warfarin is that such a regimen is likely to enhance patient compliance, a critical issue for any therapy being considered for long-term use. In contrast to full-dose warfarin which can often require weekly monitoring, low-intensity regimens have proven safe even with infrequent monitoring intervals. Further, the effect of changes in concomitant medications among patients on low-intensity warfarin is much smaller, and the risk of adverse drug interactions markedly reduced.

To date, no randomized trial of long-term low-dose warfarin in the secondary prevention of venous thrombosis has been reported. However, laboratory data suggest that such an approach may be effective. In this regard, doses of warfarin as small as 1 mg daily have been shown to reduce plasma levels of coagulation factor VII [59], and prothrombin activation assessed by prothrombin fragment F1.2 is consistently reduced among patients with a target INR as low as 1.3 to 1.6 [60]. Further, clinical thrombosis associated with indwelling venous catheters can be prevented with doses of warfarin between 1 and 2 mg daily, even among patients in whom such doses do not increase the INR above 1.3 [61, 62].

The Prevention of Recurrent Venous Thromboembolism (PREVENT) Trial

To directly address the issue of low-intensity warfarin among patients at risk for recurrent venous thrombosis, the National Heart, Lung, and Blood Institute has recently funded the Prevention of Recurrent Venous Thromboembolism (PREVENT) trial, a randomized, double-blind, placebo-controlled evaluation of low-dose warfarin to be given over a 4-year period [16]. In brief, men and women aged 30 years and over with a history of idiopathic venous thrombosis, who have completed a standard course of outpatient anticoagulation and have no contraindications to long-term therapy, will be randomly assigned to targeted low-dose warfarin (INR 1.5–2.0) which will be monitored in a double-blind manner over the course of the trial. Qualifying venous thromboembolic events must be documented by venography, compression ultrasound, ventilation-perfusion scans, magnetic resonance imaging, or pulmonary angiograms. Qualifying events must further be documented as having occurred in the absence of metastatic cancer, recent surgery, or trauma. Table 3 outlines the primary inclusion and exclusion criteria for the PREVENT trial [16].

A schematic outline of the PREVENT trial is shown in Fig. 10. All eligible patients will undergo a 28-day enrollment phase during which a stable dose of warfarin is achieved and testing for factor V Leiden will be performed. During this phase, plasma will also be obtained to evaluate for the presence of other

TABLE 3. Primary inclusion and exclusion criteria for the Prevention of Recurrent Venous Thromboembolism (PREVENT) trial

Inclusion criteria
    Documented venous thromboembolism not occurring within 90 days of surgery or trauma and have completed prescribed anticoagulation therapy within the past 2 years
    No contraindications to long-term warfarin therapy
    Age ≥ 30 years

Exclusion criteria
    History of metastatic cancer, hemorrhagic stroke, or major gastrointestinal bleeding
    Women of child-bearing potential
    Requirements for drugs that affect prothrombin time or elevated baseline international normalized ratio
    Life expectancy of less than 3 years
    Known antiphospholipid syndromes

Adapted from [16].

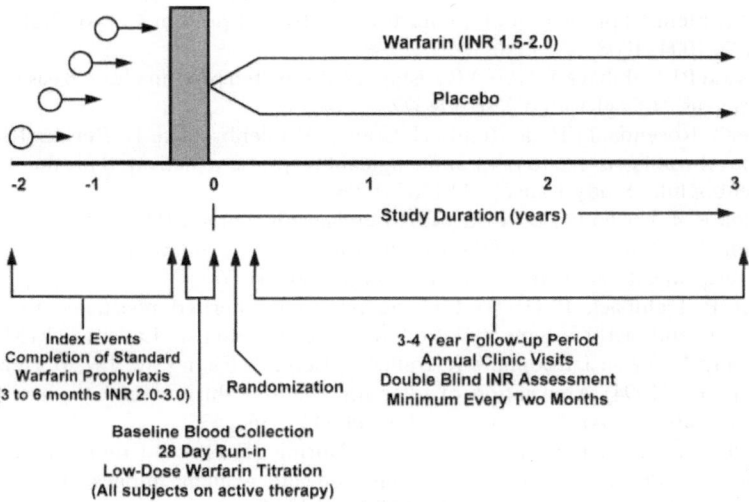

FIG. 10. Overview of the Prevention of Recurrent Venous Thromboembolism (PREVENT) trial. *INR*, international normalized ratio. (From [16], with permission)

primary hypercoagulable states. Trial endpoints will include recurrent venous-thrombosis (deep vein thrombosis and pulmonary embolism), major bleeding episodes (including hemorrhagic stroke), and all-cause mortality in the total patient population and separately in those patients who carry the factor V Leiden mutation. Reported endpoints will require full medical verification using standardized criteria based upon compression ultrasound data, ventilation-perfusion scanning, and pulmonary angiograms. During the treatment phase, all study subjects will undergo double-blind INR evaluations at least every 2 months with automated dose adjustments made to ensure a targeted INR range.

Sham dose adjustments will be made in the placebo group to ensure study blinding.

The PREVENT trial was scheduled to begin enrollment at 35 United States clinical centers by the end of 1998. The results of the PREVENT trial should provide definitive data regarding the clinical effectiveness of chronic low-dose warfarin in the secondary prevention of venous thrombosis among all patients with a prior idiopathic event, and among those at unusually high risk due to the presence of inherited defects of hemostasis such as the factor V Leiden mutation [16].

References

1. Schafer AI (1997) The primary and secondary hypercoagulable states. In: Schafer AI (ed) Molecular mechanisms of hypercoagulable states. Landes Bioscience, 1997
2. Dahlbäck B, Carlsson M, Svensson PJ (1993) Familial thrombophilia due to a previously unrecognized mechanism characterized by poor anticoagulant response to activated protein C: prediction of a cofactor to activated protein C. Proc Natl Acad Sci USA 90:1004–1008
3. Svensson PJ, Dahlbäck B (1994) Resistance to activated protein C as a basis for venous thrombosis. N Engl J Med 330:517–522
4. Koster T, Rosendaal FR, de Ronde H, Briet E, Vandenbroucke JP, Bertina RM (1993) Venous thrombosis due to poor anticoagulant response to activated protein C: Leiden Thrombophilia Study. Lancet 342:1503–1506
5. Bertina RM, Koeleman B, Koster T, Rosendaal FR, Dirven RJ, de Ronde H, van der Velden PA, Reitsma PH (1994) Mutation in blood coagulation factor V associated with resistance to activated protein C. Nature 369:64–67
6. Zoller B, Dahlbäck B (1994) Linkage between inherited resistance to activated protein C and factor V gene mutation in venous thrombosis. Lancet 343:1536–1538
7. Voorberg J, Roelse J, Koopman R, Buller H, Berends F, ten Cate JW, Mertens K, van Mourik JA (1994) Association of idiopathic venous thromboembolism with single point mutation at Arg[506] of factor V. Lancet 343:1535–1536
8. Ridker PM, Miletich JP, Hennekens CH, Buring JE (1997) Ethnic distribution of factor V Leiden among 4047 American men and women: implications for venous thromboembolism screening. JAMA 277:1305–1307
9. Rees DC, Cox M, Clegg JB (1995) World distribution of factor V Leiden. Lancet 346:1133–1134
10. Chan LC, Bourke C, Lam CK, Liu HW, Brookes S, Jenkins V, Pasi J (1996) Lack of activated protein C resistance in healthy Hong Kong chinese blood donors—correlation with absence of Arg 506 Gln mutation of factor V gene. Thromb Haemost 75:522–523
11. Fujimura H, Kambayashi J, Monden M, Kato H, Miyata T (1995) Coagulation factor V Leiden mutation may have a racial background. Thromb Haemost 74:1381
12. Ridker PM, Hennekens CH, Lindpaintner K, Stampfer MJ, Eisenberg PR, Miletich JP (1995) Mutation in the gene coding for coagulation factor V and the risk of myocardial infarction, stroke, and venous thrombosis in apparently healthy men. N Engl J Med 332:912–917
13. Ridker PM, Miletich JP, Stampfer MJ, Goldhaber SZ, Lindpaintner K, Hennekens CH (1995) Factor V Leiden and recurrent idiopathic venous thromboembolism. Circulation 92:2800–2802

14. Simioni P, Prandoni P, Lensing AWA, Scudeller A, Sardella C, Prins MH, Villalta S, Dazzi F, Girolami A (1997) The risk of recurrent venous thromboembolism in patients with an Arg506-Gln mutation in the gene for factor V (factor V Leiden). N Engl J Med 336:399–403

15. Price DT, Ridker PM (1997) Factor V Leiden mutation and the risks for thromboembolic disease: a clinical perspective. Ann Intern Med 127:895–903

16. Ridker PM for the PREVENT Investigators (1998) Long-term, low-dose warfarin among venous thrombosis patients with and without factor V Leiden mutation: rationale and design for the Prevention of Recurrent Venous Thromboembolism (PREVENT) trial. Vasc Med (1998) 3:67–73

17. Sun X, Evatt B, Griffin JH (1994) Blood coagulation factor Va abnormality associated with resistance to activated protein C in venous thrombophilia. Blood 83:3120–3125

18. De Ronde H, Bertina RM (1994) Laboratory diagnosis of APC resistance: a critical evaluation of the test and the development of diagnostic criteria. Thromb Haemost 72:880–886

19. Tosetto A, Rodeghiero F (1995) Diagnosis of APC resistance in patients on oral anticoagulants. Thromb Haemost 73:732–733

20. Cadroy Y, Sie P, Alhenc-Gelas M, Aiach M (1995) Evaluation of APC resistance in the plasma of patients with Q506 mutation of factor V (factor V Leiden) and treated with oral anticoagulants. Thromb Haemost 73:734–735

21. Gilmore G, Thom J, Baker RI (1996) Diagnosis of APC resistance in patients on standard or low molecular weight heparin. Thromb Haemost 75:267–269

22. Le DT, Griffin JH, Greengard JS, Mujumdar V, Rapaport SI (1995) Use of a generally applicable tissue factor-dependent factor V assay to detect activated protein C-resistant factor Va in patients receiving warfarin and in patients with lupus anticoagulant. Blood 85:1704–1711

23. Nathwani AC, Tuddenham EGD (1992) Epidemiology of coagulation disorders. Bailliere's Clin Haemotol 5:383–439

24. Zoller B, Svensson PJ, He X, Dahlbäck B (1994) Identification of the same factor V gene mutation in 47 out of 50 thrombosis-prone families with inherited resistance to activated protein C. J Clin Invest 94:2521–2524

25. Griffin JH, Evatt B, Wildeman C, Fernandez JA (1993) Anticoagulant protein C pathway defective in the majority of thrombophilic patients. Blood 82:1989–1993

26. Rosendaal FR, Koster T, Vandenbroucke JP, Reitsma PH (1995) High risk of thrombosis in patients homozygous for factor V Leiden (activated protein C resistance). Blood 85:1504–1508

27. Ridker PM, Glynn RJ, Miletich JP, Goldhaber SZ, Stampfer MJ, Hennekens CH (1997) Age-specific incidence rates of venous thromboembolism among carriers of factor V Leiden. Ann Intern Med 126:528–531

28. Ridker PM, Hennekens CH, Selhub J, Miletich JP, Malinow MR, Stampfer MJ (1997) Interrelation of hyperhomocyst(e)inemia, factor V Leiden, and risks of future venous thromboembolism. Circulation 95:1777–1782

29. Vandenbroucke JP, Koster T, Briet E, Reitsma PH, Bertina RM, Rosendaal FR (1994) Increased risk of venous thrombosis in oral-contraceptive users who are carriers of factor V Leiden mutation. Lancet 344:1453–1457

30. Bloemenkamp KW, Rosendaal FR, Helmerhorst FM, Buller HR, Vandenbroucke JP (1995) Enhancement by factor V Leiden mutation of risk of deep-vein thrombosis associated with oral contraceptives containing a third-generation progestagen. Lancet 346:1593–1596

31. Rintelen C, Mannhalter C, Ireland H, Lane DA, Knobl P, Lechner K, Pabinger I (1996) Oral contraceptives enhance the risk of clinical manifestation of venous thrombosis at a young age in females homozygous for factor V Leiden. Br J Haematol 93:487–490

32. Vandenbroucke JP, van der Meer FJM, Helmerhorst FM, Rosendaal FR (1996) Factor V Leiden: should we screen oral contraceptive users and pregnant women? BMJ 313:1127–1130

33. Holm J, Zoller B, Svensson P, Berntorp E, Erhardt L, Dahlbäck B (1994) Myocardial infarction associated with homozygous resistance to activated protein C. Lancet 344:952–953

34. Emmerich J, Poirier O, Evans A, Marques-Vidal, Arveiler D, Luc G, Aiach M, Cambien F (1995) Myocardial infarction, arg 506 to gln factor V mutation, and activated protein C resistance. Lancet 345:321

35. Prohaska W, Mannebach H, Schmidt M, Gleichmann U, Kleesiek K (1995) Evidence against heterozygous coagulation factor V 1691 G → A mutation with resistance to activated protein C being a risk factor for coronary artery disease and myocardial infarction. J Mol Med 73:521–524

36. Demarmels, Biasiutti F, Merlo C, Furan M, Sulzer I Binder BR, Lammle B (1995) No association of APC resistance with myocardial infarction. Blood Coagula Fibrinolysis 6:456–459

37. Halbmayer WM, Haushofer A, Schon R, Fischer M (1994) The prevalence of poor anticoagulant response to activated protein C (APC resistance) among patients suffering from stroke or venous thrombosis and among healthy subjects. Blood Coagula Fibrinolysis 5:51–57

38. Simioni P, de Ronde H, Prandoni P, Saladini M, Bertina RM, Girolami A (1995) Ischemic stroke in young patients with activated protein C resistance: a report of 3 cases belonging to three different kindreds. Stroke 26:885–890

39. Albucher JF, Guiraud-Chaumeil B, Choller F, Cadroy Y, Sie P (1996) Frequency of resistance to activated protein C due to factor V mutation in young mutation with ischemic stroke. Stroke 27:766–767

40. Rosendaal FR, Siscovick DS, Schwartz SM, Beverly RK, Psaty BM, Longstreth WT, Raghunathan TE, Koepsell TD, Reitsma PH (1997) Factor V Leiden (resistance to activated protein C) increases the risk of myocardial infarction in young women. Blood 89:2817–2821

41. Ridker PM (1997) Fibrinolytic and inflammatory markers for arterial occlusion: the evolving epidemiology of thrombosis and hemostasis. Thromb Haemost 78:53–59

42. Ridker PM, Vaughan DE, Stampfer MJ, Manson JE, Hennekens CH (1993) Endogenous tissue-type plasminogen activator and risk of myocardial infarction. Lancet 341:1165–1168

43. Ridker PM, Hennekens CH, Stampfer MJ, Manson JE, Vaughan DE (1994) Prospective study of endogenous tissue plasminogen activator and risk of stroke. Lancet 343:940–943

44. Ridker PM, Vaughan DE, Stampfer MJ, Manson JE, Shen C, Newcomer LM, Goldhaber SZ, Hennekens CH (1992) Baseline fibrinolytic state and the risk of future venous thrombosis. A prospective study of endogenous tissue-type plasminogen activator and plasminogen activator inhibitor. Circulation 85:1822–1827

45. Wilhelmsen L, Svärdsudd K, Korsan-Bengtsen K, Larsson B, Welin L, Tibblin G (1984) Fibrinogen as a risk factor for stroke and myocardial infarction. N Engl J Med 311:501–505

46. Ridker PM, Cushman M, Stampfer MJ, Tracey RP, Hennekens CH (1997) Inflammation, aspirin, and the risk of cardiovascular disease in apparently healthy men. New Engl J Med 336:973–979
47. Ridker PM, Cushman M, Stampfer MJ, Tracy RP, Hennekens CH (1998) Plasma concentration of C-reactive protein and risk of developing peripheral vascular disease. Circulation 97:425–428
48. Hirsh J (1995) The optimal duration of anticoagulation therapy for venous thromboembolism. N Engl J Med 332:1710–1711
49. Myers TM, Hull RD, Weg JG (1995) Antithrombotic therapy for venous thromboembolic disease. Chest 108:4:335S–351S
50. Schulman S, Rhedin AS, Lindmarker P, Carlsson A, Larfars G, Nicol P, Loogna E, Svensson E, Ljungberg B, Walter H et al (1995) A comparison of six weeks with six months of oral anticoagulation therapy after a first episode of venous thromboembolism. N Engl J Med 332:1661–1665
51. Prandoni P, Lensing AWA, Buller HR et al (1992) Deep-vein thrombosis and the incidence of subsequent symptomatic cancer. N Engl J Med 327:1128–1133
52. Prandoni P, Lensing A, Cogo A et al (1996) The long term clinical course of acute deep venous thrombosis. Ann Intern Med 125:1–7
53. Schulman S, Granqvist S, Holmstrom M et al (1997) The duration of oral anticoagulant therapy after a second epidose of venous thromboembolism. N Engl J Med 336:393–398
54. Fihn SD, Callahan CM, Martin DC et al for the National Consortium of Anticoagulation Clinics (1996) The risk for and severity of bleeding complications in elderly patients treated with warfarin. Ann Intern Med 124:970–979
55. Goodman SG, Langer A, Durica S et al (1994) Safety and anticoagulation effect of a low-dose combination of warfarin and aspirin in clinically stable coronary artery disease. Am J Cardiol 74:657–661
56. Coumadin Aspirin Reinfarction Study (CARS) Investigators (1997) Randomised double-blind trial of fixed low-dose warfarin with aspirin after myocardial infarction. Lancet 350:389–396
57. Meade TW, Roderick PJ, Brennan PJ, Wilkes HC, Kelleher CC (1992) Extra-cranial bleeding and other symptoms due to low dose aspirin and low intensity oral anticoagulation. Thromb Haemost 68:1–6
58. Medical Research Council's General Practice Research Framework (1998) Thrombosis prevention trial: randomised trial of low-intensity oral anticoagulation with warfarin and low-dose aspirin in the primary prevention of ischaemic heart disease in men with increased risk. Lancet 351:233–241
59. Poller L, MacCallum PK, Thomson JM, Kerns W (1990) Reduction of factor VII coagulant activity (VIIC), a risk factor for ischemic heart disease, by fixed dose warfarin: a double blind crossover study. Br Heart J 63:231–233
60. Millenson MM, Bauer KA, Kistler JP et al (1992) Monitoring "mini-intensity" anticoagulation with warfarin: comparison of the prothrombin time using a sensitive thromboplastin with prothrombin fragment F 1 + 2 levels. Blood 79:2034–2038
61. Bern MM, Likich JJ, Wallach SR et al (1990) Very low doses of warfarin can prevent thrombosis in central vein catheters. Ann Intern Med 112:423–428
62. Bern MM, Bothe A, Bistrian B et al (1986) Prophylaxis against central vein thrombosis with low-dose warfarin. Surgery 99:216–220
63. Millenson MM, Bauer KA (1996) Pathogenesis of venous thrombolembolism. In: Hull R, Pineo GF (eds) Disorders of thrombosis. WB Saunders, Philadelphia, pp 175–190

Diagnosis

Exploration of Pulmonary Embolic Sources in the Lower Limbs by Ultrasonography

SHIGETSUGU OHGI, MAROMI TACHIBANA, MASAHIKO IKEBUCHI, and YASUSHI KANAOKA

Summary. We demonstrate our method for detecting deep vein thrombosis in the lower limbs, the most frequent source of thrombosis, and we investigate the pathogenesis of critical pulmonary embolic sources. The subjects were 157 patients who underwent either pulmonary perfusion scanning or pulmonary angiography from 1987 to 1998. Unilateral thrombosis was found in 128 cases and bilateral thrombosis in 29. Among them, 42 patients exhibited symptomatic pulmonary embolism: 31 acute and 11 chronic. For exploration of deep vein thrombosis, the duplex with color Doppler was mainly used. Both sitting position and compression technique were necessary to diagnose calf vein thrombosis. Compared with the proximal occlusive levels and the incidence of symptomatic pulmonary embolism, the frequency of symptomatic pulmonary embolism was higher in the femoral vein or soleal vein than in other areas. In particular, most patients with chronic pulmonary embolism had bilateral soleal vein thrombosis. The frequency was significantly higher in bilateral thrombosis than in unilateral thrombosis. The duplex with color Doppler is the first choice of noninvasive testing methods to explore pulmonary embolic sources in the lower limbs. Both femoral vein thrombosis and soleal vein thrombosis are critical pulmonary embolic sources, and bilateral soleal vein thromboses may be a specific embolic source for chronic pulmonary embolism.

Keywords. Deep vein thrombosis, Soleal vein thrombosis, Chronic pulmonary embolism, Calf venomuscular pump, Ultrasonography

Introduction

To prevent critical pulmonary embolism in clinical practice, it is very important to diagnose an embolic source as soon as possible. However, exploration of embolic sources is difficult because the venous system is vast. Since deep vein

Second Department of Surgery, Tottori University Faculty of Medicine, 36-1 Nishi-cho, Yonago, Tottori 683-0826, Japan

thrombosis is known to occur most frequently in the lower limbs [1], a thorough exploration method should be employed even in patients with no thrombotic symptoms. The precise mechanism of transition from deep vein thrombosis to pulmonary embolism has not yet been elucidated [1, 2].

We demonstrate here our detection and evaluation methods using ultrasonography to explore pulmonary embolic sources in the lower limbs. We have investigated the specific occlusive level and pattern of thrombi as a critical embolic source.

Patients and Methods

The subjects were 157 patients diagnosed with deep vein thrombosis in the lower limb from 1987 to 1998 who underwent either pulmonary perfusion scanning or pulmonary angiography. Unilateral thrombosis was demonstrated in 128 and bilateral thrombosis in 29 patients. Their mean age was 61 years, and the male-to-female ratio was 62:95. Among them, 42 patients exhibited symptomatic pulmonary embolism: acute in 31 and chronic in 11. According to the severity of acute pulmonary embolism by the Society for Vascular Surgery, 12 patients with the acute type were in grade 1, 13 in grade 2, 4 in grade 3, and 2 in grade 4.

The patients were first diagnosed with deep vein thrombosis using ultrasonography, but venography was also performed in selected cases to confirm the diagnosis. Ultrasonic B-mode imaging with a Doppler flowmeter was performed from 1987 to 1995, and then the duplex with color Doppler was introduced in 1995.

When performing ultrasonography, we examined patients in the supine position from the inferior vena cava to the proximal popliteal segment, and then asked them to change to the sitting position, to relax the muscles and dilate the small veins in the crural region. To explore thrombi in the crural region, the distal popliteal vein was first examined at a knee-joint angle of more than 90°. Then, peroneal veins, posterior tibial veins, and the branches of soleal veins were continuously examined at the knee-joint angle of nearly 90°. In the soleal veins, poor compressibility of the vein was the most important factor to confirm thrombosis. We used a compression technique together with color flow Doppler methods (Fig. 1). At first, we carefully observed blood flow regarding the presence of echogenic thrombi without comperssion. Then, we confirmed the size of thrombi with light compression. Finally, we evaluated the consistency of the thrombi with moderate compression.

Patients with symptomatic pulmonary embolism were mainly diagnosed using perfusion scanning according to the Prospective Investigation of Pulomonary Embolism Diagnosis [3], and ventilation scanning and/or angiography were performed in selected severe cases. In patients without symptoms of pulmonary embolism, interpretation of pulmonary perfusion was judged as normal or abnormal.

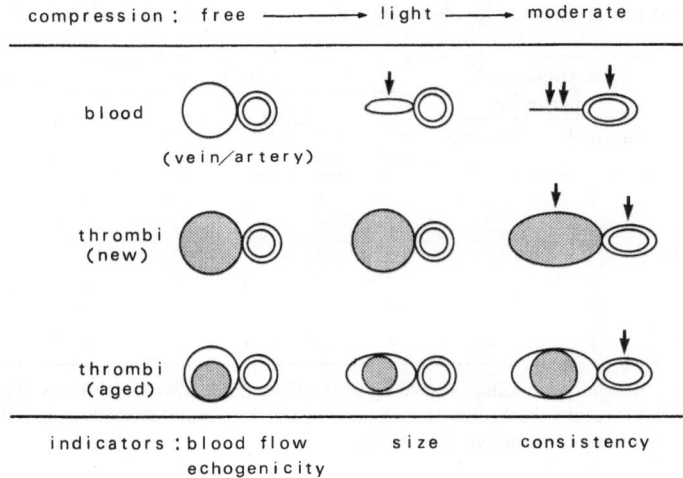

FIG. 1. Our detection and evaluation methods for venous thrombi by ultrasonography

TABLE 1. Proximal occlusive levels and pulmonary embolism in unilateral deep vein thrombosis

Location	No.	Asymptomatic perfusion		Symptomatic					Total no. (%)
				Acute				Chronic	
		normal	abnormal	G-1	G-2	G-3	G-4		
Iliac	75	42	24	6	2	1	–	–	9 (12)
Femoral	17	4	2	2	4	1	1	3	11 (65)
Popliteal	12	4	5	1	2	–	–	–	3 (25)
Crural	2	2	–	–	–	–	–	–	0 (0)
Soleal	22	14	2	3	3	–	–	–	6 (27)
Case no.	128	66	33	12	11	2	1	3	29 (23)

G-1–4; grade of pulmonary embolism according to the Society for Vascular Surgery [4].

Results

Proximal Occlusive Levels and Pulmonary Embolism

In patients with unilateral deep vein thrombosis, the relationship between the proximal occlusive levels and the pulmonary embolism was analyzed (Table 1). Although the frequency of proximal occlusive levels was higher in the iliac veins than those in other veins, the frequency rate of symptomatic pulmonary embolism was the highest in the femoral vein.

In patients with bilateral deep vein thrombosis, the relationship between the proximal occlusive levels and the pulmonary embolism was also analyzed (Table 2). The frequency of proximal occlusive levels was higher in the soleal veins than

TABLE 2. Proximal occlusive levels and pulmonary embolism in bilateral deep vein thrombosis

Location	No.	Asymptomatic perfusion		Symptomatic					Total no. (%)
				Acute				Chronic	
		normal	abnormal	G-1	G-2	G-3	G-4		
Iliac	14	7	2	2	1	2	–	–	5 (36)
Femoral	12	5	2	2	1	2	–	–	5 (42)
Popliteal	4	4	–	–	–	–	–	–	0 (0)
Crural	3	–	–	–	–	–	1[a]	2[a]	3 (100)
Soleal	25	8	2	–	–	–	1	14	15 (60)
Total no.	58	24	6	4	2	4	2	16	28 (48)*

G-1–4; grade of pulmonary embolism according to the Society for Vascular Surgery [4].
[a] Three patients with soleal vein thromboses on one leg and with crural thromboses on the other leg. These patients are excluded from Tables 3 and 4.
* $P < 0.01$.

in other veins, and the frequency of symptomatic pulmonary embolism was highest in the crural veins followed by the soleal veins.

The frequency of symptomatic pulmonary embolism in patients with bilateral thrombosis was significantly higher than that of patients with unilateral thrombosis.

Specific Proximal Occlusive Patterns of Critical Embolic Sources

The proximal occlusive pattern 1 in the femoral vein is shown in Fig. 2. This patient was diagnosed as having chronic pulmonary embolism with severe pulmonary hypertension, but did not have any symptoms of deep vein thrombosis in either lower limb. However, ultrasonography revealed visible proximal thrombi in the left distal common femoral vein propagating from the crural veins.

The proximal occlusive pattern 2 in the soleal vein is shown in Fig. 3. This patient was diagnosed as having chronic pulmonary embolism with severe pulmonary hypertension, but did not have any symptoms of deep vein thrombosis in either lower limb. However, ultrasonography revealed isolated thrombi in the central branches of the bilateral soleal veins.

Extent of Soleal Vein Thrombosis and Pulmonary Embolism

In 33 patients with soleal vein thrombosis, the relationship between the extent of thrombosis and pulmonary embolism was analyzed (Table 3). The main central branch was the most frequent site of soleal vein thrombosis. Among the patients with symptomatic pulmonary embolism, all but one demonstrated thrombosed central branches of soleal veins.

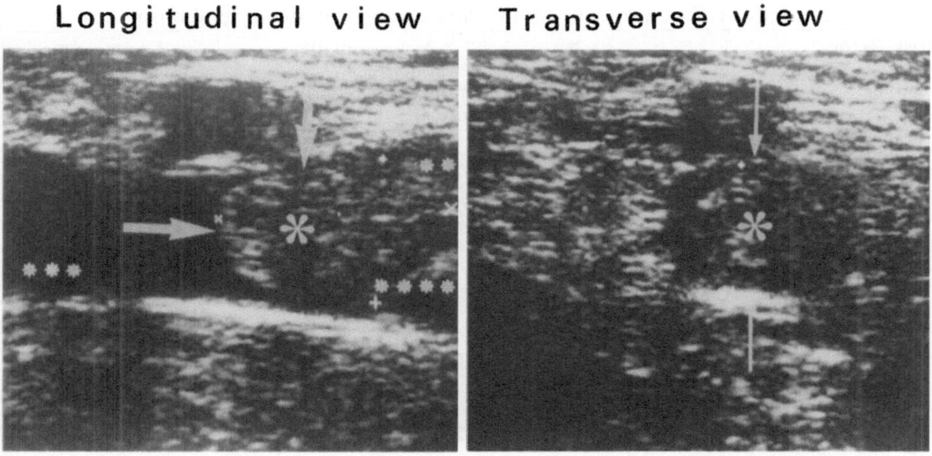

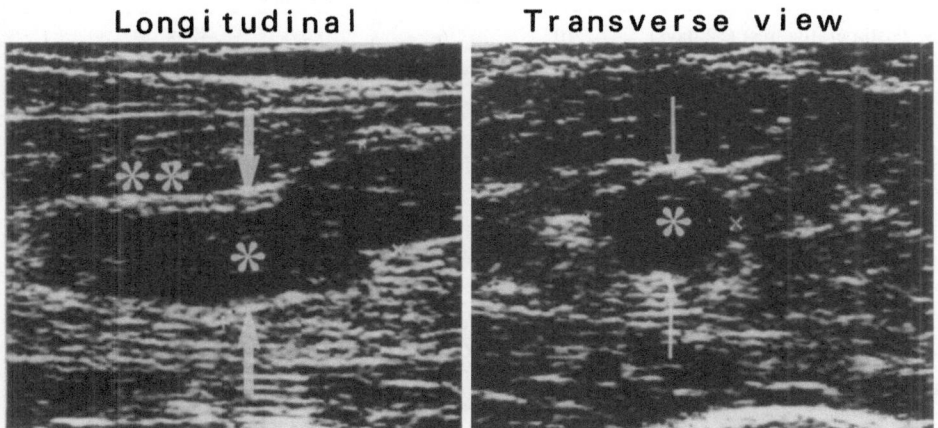

Longitudinal view   Transverse view

FIG. 2. Proximal occlusive pattern 1 in the left distal common femoral vein. *Visible echogenic thrombi; **superficial femoral vein; ***common femoral vein; ****deep femoral vein

Longitudinal   Transverse view

FIG. 3. Proximal occlusive pattern 2 in the central branches of the bilateral soleal veins. *Nonvisible echogenic thrombi; **soleal vein

TABLE 3. Extent of isolated soleal vein thrombosis and pulmonary embolism

Risk factor	No.	Asymptomatic perfusion		Symptomatic	
		normal	abnormal	acute	chronic
Single branch					
central	22	14	2	3	3
medial	6	4	1	1	–
lateral	1	1	–	–	–
Two branches					
centromedial	7	2	–	1	4
centrolateral	4	–	–	1	3
mediolateral	–	–	–	–	–
Three branches	3	–	1	–	2
Total no. of limbs	43	21	4	6	12

TABLE 4. Risk factors of isolated soleal vein thrombosis and pulmonary embolism

Risk factor	No.	Asymptomatic perfusion		Symptomatic	
		normal	abnormal	acute	chronic
1. Postoperative rest (>2 days)	10	6	–	3	1
2. Other bed rest (>2 days)	3	1	2	–	–
3. Thrombophilia	1	1	–	–	–
4. Drug	3	2	–	–	1
5. Malignancy	2	2	–	–	–
6. Primary varicose vein	10	6	2	1	1
7. Unknown	4	–	–	1	3
Total no. of patients	33	18	4	5	6

Risk Factors of Soleal Vein Thrombosis and Pulmonary Embolism

The relationship between risk factors of soleal vein thrombosis and pulmonary embolism was analyzed (Table 4). Postoperative immobility and varicose veins are possible risk factors for soleal vein thrombosis, but there were no significant risk factors for the pulmonary embolism.

Critical Pulmonary Embolism Based on Soleal Vein Thrombosis

During a 7-year period, we found nine critical patients, one acute and eight chronic, based on soleal vein thrombosis. All eight patients with the chronic pulmonary embolism demonstrated bilateral soleal vein thrombosis. Rapid type

TABLE 5. Chronic pulmonary embolism based on bilateral soleal vein thromboses

Type	Age (years)	Sex	Term	NYHA grade	AB	PaO$_2$ (mmHg)	PSS	PAG	mPA (mmHg)
Rapid									
Case 1	53	M	1 week	3	n	62	l	+	84/32 (52)
Case 2	49	F	2 week	3	ANA	57	d	+	94/38 (58)
Case 4	37	F	1 month	4	LAC	–	m	+	73/24 (42)
Case 3	78	F	3 week	4	–	46	m	+	80/30 (50)
Slow									
Case 5	78	F	2 years	1	RA	58	d	+	53/8 (30)
Case 6	51	F	2 years	3	n	58	m	–	75/35 (50)
Case 7	56	M	6 months	3	–	66	m	+	103/29 (58)
Case 8	61	F	2 years	3	RA, ANA	45	m	+	112/34 (59)

NYHA, New York Heart Association; AB, serum antibody; PSS, pulmonary perfusion scanning; PAG, pulmonary angiography; mPA, mean pulmonary artery pressure; n, normal; ANA, antinuclear antibody; LAC, lupus anticoagulant; RA, rheumatoid factor; l, local; d, diffuse; m, multiple.

patients in whom the duration of disease was less than 3 months differed from slow patients (Table 5). All rapid type patients had severe pulmonary hypertension greater than 40 mmHg of mean pulmonary arterial pressure, but one of the four type patients had moderate hypertension.

Discussion

Exploration of Pulmonary Embolic Sources

Two situations exist regarding exploration for pulmonary embolic sources: patients with pulmonary embolism both with symptoms of deep vein thrombosis and without symptoms of deep vein thrombosis [1]. In the latter group, extensive exploration is mandatory to begin treatment for reliable prevention of recurrent pulmonary embolism and all general venous systems must be examined as possible embolic sources. However, the venous system in the lower limbs should be examined first using noninvasive screening tests. In the former group, standard exploration is important for secondary prevention, and symptomatic venous systems mainly in the lower limbs must be examined as probable embolic sources.

Among the many methods for exploration, the duplex has been the first choice for detecting venous thrombi in the lower limbs [1, 5, 6]. Our diagnostic accuracy of ultrasonography is summarized in Table 6 [7, 8]. To diagnose venous thrombi with duplex scanning, the noncompressible venous space is reliably confirmed using the compression technique. Evaluation of blood flow is also necessary for venous obstruction or insufficiency. When using the compression technique in the crural region, patients should be kept in the sitting position, because it is very

TABLE 6. Diagnostic accuracy of ultrasonography in deep vein thrombosis in the lower limbs

Location	Sensitivity (%)	Specificity (%)	Total accuracy (%)
Common iliac vein	75	100	90
External iliac vein	89	100	92
Common femoral vein	100	100	100
Superficial femoral vein	84	–	94
Popliteal vein	100	100	100
Posterior tibial vein	11	97	82
Anterior tibial vein	–	–	–
Peroneal vein	83	98	96
Soleal vein	95	96	98
Gastrocnemial vein	33	100	96

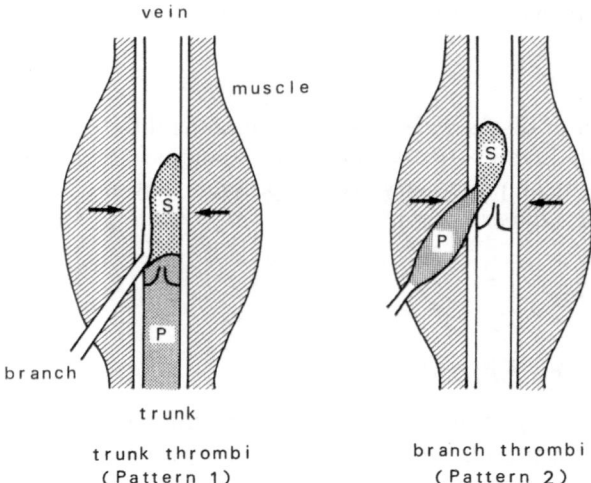

trunk thrombi
(Pattern 1)

branch thrombi
(Pattern 2)

FIG. 4. Productive mechanism of critical pulmonary emboli in the lower limbs

difficult to confirm venous thrombi in small veins unless maximal venous dilatation are maintained. On the other hand, in the thoracic or abdominal large veins, computerized tomography or magnetic resonance imaging is very effective for screening venous thrombi.

Pathogenesis of Embolic Sources in Critical Pulmonary Embolism

There are three main processes for the transition from deep vein thrombosis to pulmonary embolisms (Fig. 4). Primary or secondary thrombi may become emboli because of lower limb movement.

TABLE 7. Recurrent productive mechanism of emboli in specific locations of the lower limbs

	Pattern 1	Pattern 2
1. Location	Femoral vein	Soleal vein
2. Mechanism	Detach	Expel
3. Cause	Compression	Calf muscle pump
4. Activity	Limb movement (supine)	Walking

We analyzed the relationship between the proximal level of thrombi and the frequency of pulmonary embolic symptoms. Since both femoral and soleal levels had higher frequencies of pulmonary embolism than other sources, they are considered critical embolic sources. We further analyzed the precise occlusive patterns in both levels. The femoral level had patent proximal common femoral and iliac veins, and the soleal level had patent soleal veins and proximal crural veins. From these results, we propose that the secondary thrombi in the proximal common femoral vein are detached by compression due to limb movement in any position. On the other hand, the secondary thrombi in the soleal veins are expelled by the calf muscle pump due to walking (Table 7). Since these productive mechanisms may be repeated by daily activity, pulmonary vasculature may deteriorate according to both the speed and frequency of embolic reccurrence.

Critical Pulmonary Embolism Based on Soleal Vein Thrombosis

The soleal vein may be a special location for deep vein thrombosis in the lower limbs [1, 9]. It is unknown whether this vein plays a role in deep vein thrombosis or pulmonary embolism. We also reported that soleal vein thrombosis occurred most frequently in the calf vein thromboses [8]. Since soleal vein thrombosis occurred most frequently in the central branch, this main large branch is possibly an origin of calf vein thrombosis. Postoperative immobility may be a risk factor, but dilatation of the soleal vein might be related to thrombosis.

Calf vein thrombosis containing soleal vein thrombosis has not been widely accepted as a critical embolic source [2, 10]. Within a 7-year period, we observed acute or chronic critical pulmonary embolism in 12 patients with soleal vein thrombosis, most of whom had no symptoms of deep vein thrombosis [8]. The pathogenesis of chronic pulmonary embolism is still unknown. We found eight patients with pulmonary hypertension who had bilateral soleal vein thromboses. However, patients with unilateral soleal vein thrombosis did not demonstrate chronic pulmonary embolism but did exhibit acute pulmonary embolism. Therefore, bilateral soleal vein thrombosis may be a specific embolic source of chronic pulmonary embolism. As mentioned above, since soleal veins are a main component of the calf pump, daily walking may produce recurrent emboli.

Conclusion

Duplex with color Doppler is the initial noninvasive test for exploration of pulmonary embolic sources in the lower limbs. Both femoral vein and soleal veins are critical pulmonary embolic sources. Bilateral soleal vein thromboses seem to be a specific source for chronic pulmonary embolism.

References

1. Browse NL, Burnand KG, Lea Thomas M (1988) Diseases of the vein. Edward Arnold, London, pp 581–594
2. Kistner RL, Ball JJ, Nordyke RA et al (1972) Incidence of pulmonary embolism in the course of thrombophlebitis of the lower extremities. Am J Surg 124:169–176
3. The PIOPED investigators (1991) Value of the ventilation/perfusion scan in acute pulmonary embolism. Results of the prospective investigation of pulmonary embolism diagnosis (PIOPED). JAMA 263:2753–2759
4. Porter JM, Rutherford RB, Clagett GP et al (1988) Reporting standards in venous disease. J Vasc Surg 8:172–181
5. Cranley JJ (1990) Diagnosis of deep vein thrombosis. In: Bernstein EF (ed) Noninvasive diagnostic techniques in vascular disease. Mosby, St. Louis, pp 207–212
6. Talbot SR (1986) B-mode evaluation of peripheral arteries and veins. In: Zwiebel WJ (ed) Introduction to vascular ultrasonography. Grune and Stratton, Orlando, pp 351–383
7. Ohgi S, Tanaka K, Ito K et al (1989) Diagnosis of deep vein thrombosis by high resolutional ultrasonography. J Jpn Surg Soc 91:424–430
8. Ohgi S, Tachibana M, Ikebuchi M et al (1998) Pulmonary embolism in patients with isolated soleal vein thrombosis. Angiology 49:759–764
9. Browse NL, Lea Thomas M (1974) Source of non-lethal pulmonary emboli. Lancet 1:258–289
10. Gachino A (1988) Relationship between deep vein thrombosis and the calf and fetal pulmonary embolism. Can J Surg 31:129–130

Echocardiography in Pulmonary Embolism

Scott D. Solomon

Summary. Echocardiography has emerged as an important and unique diagnostic tool in patients with acute pulmonary embolism (PE). In addition to occasionally providing direct visualization of thrombus within the right-sided chambers and pulmonary arteries, echocardiography provides crucial information about cardiac function, particularly the function of the right ventricle. Exquisitely sensitive to changes in afterload, a previously normal right ventricle dilates and becomes dysfunctional in the setting of PE. Indeed, we have identified a specific pattern of right ventricular regional wall motion that is often present in patients with PE. In addition to providing important diagnostic information, these alterations in right ventricular morphology and function provide prognostic information as well, as patients who have evidence of right ventricular dysfunction have a higher incidence of death and recurrent PE. Echocardiography can be used to identify patients at high risk following PE and thus can be used to identify those patients who would most benefit from aggressive therapies, including thrombolysis, and open or suction embolectomy. Finally, echocardiography provides a unique insight into the pathophysiology of PE and the function of the right ventricle in pulmonary vascular disease.

Keywords. Pulmonary embolism, Echocardiography, Right ventricle, Diagnosis, Prognosis

Introduction

Pulmonary embolism (PE) continues to be a significant cause of morbidity and mortality in hospitalized and nonhospitalized patients with estimates of approximately 50 000 deaths per year in the United States [1]. Traditional methods for diagnosing PE include isotope-based ventilation-perfusion scanning or pulmonary angiography. Currently, a number of therapeutics option exist for

Cardiovascular Division, Brigham and Women's Hospital, 75 Francis Street, Boston, MA 02115, USA patients with acute PE, including traditional therapies such as simple anticoagulation and inferior vena cava filter placement, and more aggressive approaches, such as thrombolysis, open embolectomy, and catheter-based suction embolectomy. Despite much improvement over the past decade in the diagnosis and management of patients with PE, this diagnosis continues to elude clinicians in the complicated patient population in which the diagnosis is most common and is competing with other cardiovascular and pulmonary conditions that often coexist. The existence of new therapeutics options for treating acute PE makes it essential to have the ability to identify the highest risk patients who would most benefit from the most aggressive therapies.

Echocardiography has emerged as a diagnostic test of significant value in patients with acute PE, providing diagnostic, functional, and prognostic information. In addition, echocardiography has provided unique insights into the function of the right ventricle in the setting of PE. This paper will review the utility of echocardiography in the diagnosis of PE, the pathophysiologic insights that echocardiography offers in the setting of PE, and the prognostic information that echocardiography provides.

Echocardiography for the Diagnosis and Direct Visualization of Thrombus

Thrombi that are responsible for pulmonary emboli most commonly form in the deep veins of the legs and embolize to the pulmonary arteries. Nevertheless, thrombus can form anywhere in the venous system, including the pelvic veins, vena cavae, right atrium, right ventricle and, under rare circumstances, the pulmonary arteries and arterioles themselves. Echocardiography has proven useful in visualization of thrombi in a number of these locations. Kasper et al. identified intraluminal filling defects in 13 out of 105 patients (12%) with clinical or postmortem diagnosis of PE [2]. These defects included right pulmonary artery thrombus in 11 patients and right ventricular thrombus in 3 patients. In addition, thrombi have been reported in numerous series and case reports in the superior vena cava, the innominate vein, the right atrium, and the inferior vena cava [3–5]. While thrombi visualized in locations other than the pulmonary arteries are not themselves diagnostic of PE, these findings are extremely useful when identified because they significantly enhance the suspicion of this diagnosis when the clinical scenario is appropriate. In most reported cases of right-sided thrombi, acute or recurrent pulmonary emboli were observed.

Transthoracic echocardiography (TTE) is extremely useful in the diagnosis of thrombus in the vena caval—right atrial junction, the right atrium, the right ventricle, the right ventricular outflow tract, and the proximal pulmonary arteries. Generally, TTE can effectively visualize the pulmonary arteries to the level of the bifurcation, although the ability to visualize even the bifurcation can be compromised in patients with poor echocardiographic windows. Thrombi that form within the deep veins of the legs tend to be long and wormlike, and can be visualized in transit and as saddle emboli. Thrombi that form within the right-sided chambers themselves are more likely globular or mural in morphology. These often need to be distinguished from tumor, myxoma, and other pathologic conditions that can resemble thrombi. Nevertheless, nonthrombotic lesions in the right-sided chambers, including right-sided vegetations and myxoma, have also been associated with pulmonary embolic disease.

More recently, the improved imaging quality of transesophageal echocardiography (TEE) has proved useful in the visualization of pulmonary emboli. Although TEE does not offer a significant advantage over TTE for visualizing the right ventricle and atrium, TEE visualization of the pulmonary arteries themselves is improved over TTE, usually at least a few centimeters beyond the pulmonary bifurcation. Yet despite the improved resolution of TEE, this technique is rarely used as the primary means to diagnose PE. The reason for this is twofold: although the identification of pulmonary artery thrombi certainly substantiates the diagnosis of PE, the inability to visualize much beyond the pulmonary bifurcation greatly limits the sensitivity of this technique. Second, the requirement for conscious sedation in patients undergoing TEE may be impractical in the setting of acute pulmonary compromise, and is virtually contraindicated in nonintubated patients in whom oxygen saturation is less than 90%. More often, the diagnosis will be made on TEE performed for other reasons, usually to rule out other cardiovascular causes of pulmonary compromise, even when the diagnosis of PE is not suspected. Unfortunately, the true incidence of visualized thrombi in patients with suspected PE is unknown but likely is under 20%. The incidence of thrombi in the pulmonary arteries themselves is considerably lower. This low incidence makes either technique—TTE or TEE—impractical as a primary means to diagnose PE. Clinically, it is important to recognize that these findings, when present, certainly contribute to the diagnosis of PE, but when absent do not rule out the possibility of PE (see Fig. 1).

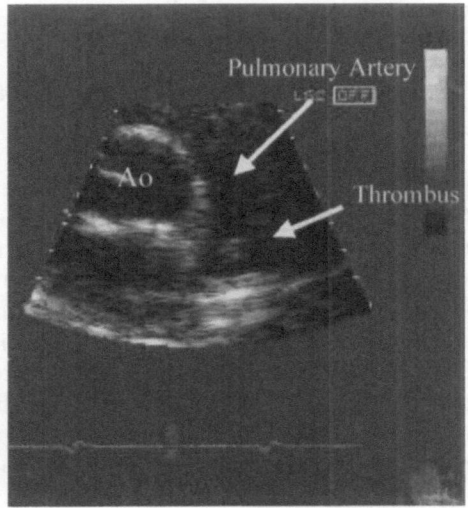

FIG. 1. Short-axis echocardiographic image through the base of the heart showing a thrombus visualized in the pulmonary artery at the level of the pulmonary bifurcation. *Ao*, aorta

Diagnosis of Pulmonary Artery Abnormalities and Pulmonary Hypertension

Other abnormalities of the pulmonary arteries can be visualized with either transthoracic or transesophageal echocardiography in the setting of PE. Increases in pulmonary arterial size can be seen with echocardiography and can indicate acute elevations in pulmonary resistance [6]. In addition, pulmonic regurgitation, while commonly seen in normal patients, can be significant in PE. Doppler examination of either pulmonic regurgitation or tricuspid regurgitation can provide direct evidence of elevated pulmonary pressures. The end-diastolic pulmonic regurgitant velocity reflects the difference between end-diastolic pulmonary pressure and end-diastolic right ventricular pressures. Utilizing the modified Bernoulli equation, $P = 4 \times V^2$, and adding a bedside estimate of right atrial pressure yields an estimate of pulmonary diastolic pressures. Similarly, the velocity of tricuspid regurgitation reflects the pressure gradient between the right ventricle and the right atrium in systole, and this estimate, also utilizing the modified Bernoulli equation, added to right atrial pressure yields an estimate of pulmonary artery systolic pressure. Nevertheless, while the extent of tricuspid regurgitation visualized on color flow Doppler examination can be increased in the setting of PE, the velocity of tricuspid regurgitation, reflective of the pulmonary pressures, may not be—and is often not—increased. This is because a normal right ventricle, when faced with elevated pulmonary resistance, cannot generate significantly higher systolic pressures acutely. In contrast, however, patients with long-standing pulmonary vascular disease of any etiology, including recurrent or chronic pulmonary emboli, will demonstrate elevations of pulmonary pressure identified by echocardiography. Commonly, these patients will also have evidence of right ventricular hypertrophy. These findings can be useful in the diagnosis of long-standing pulmonary vascular disease, but cannot distinguish between the myriad of causes of pulmonary hypertension and specifically cannot diagnose chronic pulmonary emboli.

The Right Ventricle in Pulmonary Embolism

The pathophysiologic effect of acute PE is to cause an acute abrupt increase in pulmonary vascular resistance. The process by which this effect occurs is twofold: first, pulmonary emboli result in mechanical occlusion of a portion of the pulmonary vasculature. This, in turn, results in increased flow in other regions of the vasculature with a direct elevation of pulmonary resistance. In addition, further increases in pulmonary vascular resistance occur with the release of vasoconstricting factors such as serotonin, with reflex vasoconstriction and with hypoxemia-induced vasoconstriction after acute PE [7]. Increased pulmonary vascular resistance results in increased load on the right ventricle but does not result in marked elevations in pulmonary artery pressure. Indeed, in patients with angiographic obstruction ranging from 13% to 68%, mean pulmonary pressures never exceeded 40 mmHg [8]. Patients in whom angiographic obstruction was less than 30% generally did not have increased pulmonary pressures. In these studies, however, baseline pulmonary pressures were unknown, and the extent to which these patients may have had some degree of prior pulmonary hypertension is unknown.

There are a number of pathophysiologic mechanisms for the changes that occur in the right ventricle following PE. First, this acute change in load on the right ventricle results in an abrupt and marked decrease in right ventricular fractional shortening. If the rise in afterload is great enough, the right ventricle begins to fail, dilates, and becomes dysfunctional. Indeed, a previously normal right ventricle cannot generate sufficient pressures to overcome the increase in pulmonary vascular resistance. Right ventricular pressures rise only minimally, with resulting right ventricular dilatation and the appearance of right ventricular dysfunction. Nevertheless, the overall contractile state of the right ventricle may not change. Rather, the healthy right ventricular muscle demonstrates marked reduction in fractional shorting when subjected to a load greater than it can accommodate. In the worst cases, this can lead to failure of the right ventricle.

In addition to the passive effects of the increased load on the right ventricle, ischemia may play an important role in right ventricular pathophysiology in the setting of PE. Elevations in right ventricular wall stress occur as the right ventricle dilates, and these increases in wall stress, in turn, lead to increased right ventricular oxygen demand [9]. Coronary blood flow to the right ventricle, while increased with subcritical pulmonary artery obstruction [10], may decrease in the setting of massive elevations of right-sided wall tension, or systemic hypotension. The most compelling evidence that right ventricular ischemia may be, at least in part, responsible for changes in right ventricular function during PE is derived from animal data showing that augmentation of right coronary artery flow could reverse right ventricular dysfunction in experimental PE [9]. Finally, the pathophysiologic effects that lead to ischemia can also, in extreme cases, lead to right ventricular infarction [11]. Elevations in creatine kinase (CK) with MB isoenzymes and right-sided electrocardiographic abnormalities have been observed in patients with diagnosed PE. In one study, 4 out of 52 patients with acute PE were identified who had elevations in CK-MB and evidence of right ventricular dysfunction by echocardiography [12]. The extent to which occult right coronary artery disease contributes to these findings in patients with PE is not known.

While the previously normal right ventricle responds to acute increases in pulmonary vascular resistance with dilatation and dysfunction, the response differs markedly in the right ventricle that has previously been exposed to higher pulmonary pressures. This situation occurs in patients with pulmonary hypertension of any etiology, including prior recurrent or chronic pulmonary emboli. In these cases, chronic increases in pulmonary resistance lead to hypertrophy of the right ventricle, enabling the right ventricle to generate higher pressures. The hypertrophied right ventricle is better equipped to overcome the increases in pulmonary vascular resistance associated with acute PE without failing, dilating, and becoming dysfunctional.

Echocardiographic Assessment of Right Ventricular Function in Pulmonary Embolism

Echocardiography provides unique diagnostic and prognostic information in patients with acute PE. The most important information obtained from echocardiography in the setting of acute PE is right ventricular size and function. Both of these measures provide a unique window into the pathophysiology of PE in addition to providing invaluable diagnostic and prognostic information.

The extent of echocardiographic abnormalities in PE depends largely on the extent of pulmonary blood flow that is compromised. While small pulmonary emboli can be associated with virtually no abnormalities seen on echocardiography, the majority of pulmonary emboli that are clinically detectable are associated with echocardiographic abnormalities. Indeed, various series have reported right ventricular dilatation in between 75% and 90% of patients with PE [2, 13]. In the adult, the right ventricular diameter in the apical four-chamber view (Fig. 2) is between 0.9 and 2.6 cm, with a mean of 1.9 cm [14]. In contrast, the mean right ventricular diameter in PE has been reported to be greater than 2.7 cm [2, 15]. Indeed, right ventricular diameter has been correlated with the degree of vascular obstruction ($r = 0.8$) in patients with no prior history of cardiopulmonary disease [15]. Since normally the right ventricular diameter in the apical four-chamber view is substantially less that left ventricular diameter in this view, we have generally considered the right ventricle to be dilated if right ventricular diameter in the apical four-chamber view exceeds left ventricular diameter. This simple assessment obviates the need for making actual measurements of the right ventricle, but is limited to patients in whom the left ventricle itself is not dilated. Finally, the most common causes of right ventricular dilatation that need to be distinguished from PE include right ventricular infarction, congestive heart

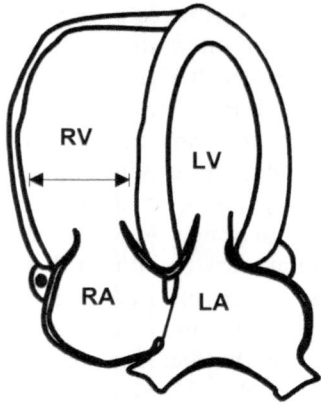

Fig. 2. Schematic drawing of apical four-chamber view. The correct location for measurement of the right ventricular diameter is shown (*arrows*). *RA*, right atrium; *RV*, right ventricle; *LA*, left atrium; *LV*, left ventriale

failure, chronic tricuspid regurgitation, pulmonary stenosis, and atrial septal defect.

Although right ventricular dilatation represents the most common echocardiographic finding in PE, it is the constellation of echocardiographic findings in acute PE that makes echocardiography an important diagnostic and prognostic tool. Echocardiographic findings associated with acute PE are shown in Table 1. The most striking echocardiographic abnormality in acute PE is right ventricular dilatation and dysfunction. As mentioned previously, the normal right ventricle, when subjected to an increased load, will dilate and begin to fail. By echocardiography, right ventricular failure is most commonly appreciated as decreased wall motion excursion in the right ventricular free wall. These abnormalities are usually best visualized in the apical four-chamber views. Indeed, the complex crescent-like shape of the right ventricle makes echocardiographic visualization considerably more difficult than the left ventricle. Parasternal short and long axis images of the right ventricle are difficult to standardize and interpret. Finally, the heavy trabeculation of the right ventricle makes endocardial wall definition difficult. M-Mode measurements of the right ventricle are considerably less commonly used than in the past, and in our laboratory, we have relied almost solely on two-dimensional assessments of the right ventricle.

Left Ventricular Function in Pulmonary Embolism

In contrast to the right ventricle, left ventricular function may be normal or even increased in PE. Pulmonary vascular obstruction does reduce left ventricular preload, leading to the echocardiographic appearance of an underfilled left ventricle. In addition, increased sympathetic tone and neurohormonal changes are associated with both tachycardia and hypercontractility of the left ventricle. The finding of right ventricular dilatation and dysfunction in the setting of normal or hyperdynamic left ventricular function should always strongly raise the suspicion for PE, and help distinguish PE from other causes of right ventricular dysfunction and dilatation.

TABLE 1. Echocardiographic findings in acute pulmonary embolism

Right ventricular dilatation
Right ventricular dysfunction (regional, see text)
Normal or hyperdynamic left ventricular function
Paradoxic septal motion
Interventricular septal flattening
Tricuspid regurgitation
Pulmonary artery dilatation
Attenuation of normal inspiratory collapse of inferior vena cava
Decrease in right ventricular fractional area change

Regional Right Ventricular Function in Pulmonary Embolism

While PE is associated with decreased global right ventricular function, the dysfunction that occurs is clearly of a regional nature and can be clearly appreciated by echocardiography. We have quantified this regional right ventricular dysfunction both qualitatively and quantitatively using the centerline method that is commonly utilized to assess left ventricular function [16]. In this study, regional right ventricular function was assessed qualitatively by three experienced independent echocardiographers. In addition, the right ventricular free wall in the apical four-chamber view was digitized in both systole and diastole, and chords were drawn by computer between the diastolic and systolic contours (Fig. 3). A unique pattern of regional wall motion was seen in both qualitative and quantitative analysis in which the mid-right ventricular free wall was akinetic or dyskinetic, and the apex and base of the right ventricle were normal or hyperkinetic (Fig. 4). This motion is illustrated in Fig. 5. This unusual pattern of wall motion, called McConnell's sign, can be easily appreciated on echocardiography. This pattern was defined on one group of patients and then tested on a separate validation cohort of 85 patients with right ventricular dysfunction from a broad range of etiologies. The pattern of wall motion abnormality, with normal right ventricular apical wall motion and abnormal wall motion in the mid-right ventricular free wall had a sensitivity of 77% and a specificity of 94% for PE, with a positive predictive value of 76% and a negative predictive value of 96% for an overall diagnostic accuracy of 92%. In our laboratory, we have been so convinced that this specific pattern of regional right ventricular dysfunction represents a finding unique to pulmonary embolism that we have considered this finding to be *diagnostic of PE until proven otherwise* and have urged clinicians to actively pursue the diagnosis of PE when this abnormality is recognized. (Patients with

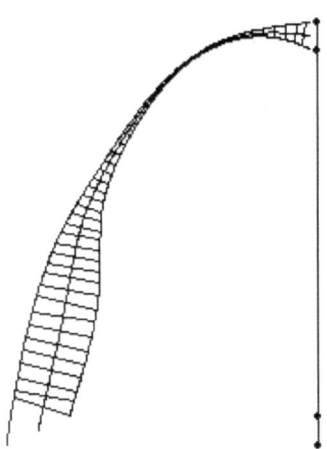

FIG. 3. Centerline method for assessing regional wall motion excursion. The right ventricular endocardium is digitized at end-diastole (*outer contour*) and end-systole (*inner contour*). The interventricular septum is represented as a straight line. Equally spaced chords are drawn by computer between the end-diastolic and end-systolic contours

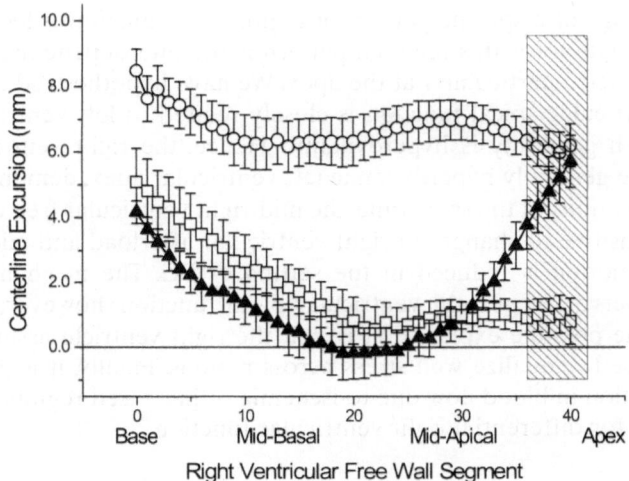

Fig. 4. Wall motion excursion (in mm) in normal controls (*open circles*), patients with primary pulmonary hypertension (*open squares*), and patients with acute pulmonary embolism (*closed triangles*). Chords are displayed along the *x*-axis from the base to the apex. The *hatched area* represents statistically significant differences between the pulmonary embolism (*PE*) patients and those with primary pulmonary hypertension. (From with permission)

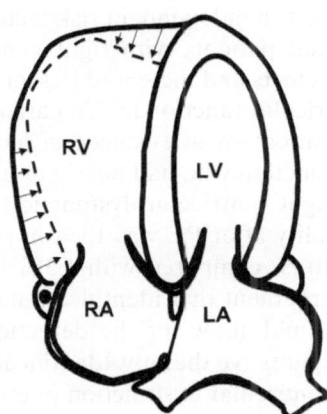

Fig. 5. Schematic showing the pattern of regional dysfunction in patients with PE. Wall motion is preserved at the apex and base, but markedly diminished in the mid-right ventricle

primary pulmonary hypertension demonstrated similar wall motion abnormalities at the base and mid-right ventricular free wall, although right ventricular wall motion remained abnormal at the apex in patients with primary pulmonary hypertension.)

While alterations in global right ventricular function in PE can be explained by the inability of the right ventricle to accommodate the acute increase in afterload, the etiology of a specific pattern of regional dysfunction is less clear. One possible explanation for this regional pattern is the interdependence of the left and right ventricles, particularly at the apex. We have hypothesized that in acute PE, right ventricular apical function is closely related to left ventricular apical function, which generally is hyperdynamic. Hence, the right ventricular apex, tethered to the generally hyperdynamic left ventricular apex, demonstrates augmented wall motion. At the same time, the mid-right ventricular free wall appears to be most sensitive to changes in right ventricular afterload and mid-right ventricular wall motion is reduced in the setting of PE. The mechanism for the observed preservation of right ventricular basal function, however, is less well explained. One possible explanation is that the right ventricle assumes a more spherical shape to equalize wall stress across regions. Finally, it is possible that regional variation in blood flow due to ischemia or increased regional wall stress is responsible for differential right ventricular function.

Prognostic Implications of Echocardiography in Pulmonary Embolism

In addition to aiding in the diagnosis of PE, echocardiography provides important prognostic information as well. In a randomized trial of thrombolysis versus heparin for PE, Goldhaber et al. demonstrated that right ventricular dysfunction was an independent risk factor for recurrent PE [17]. Similarly, Wolfe et al. found that patients with right ventricular dysfunction had both increased perfusion defects and increased risk of recurrent PE [18]. Ribeiro et al. assessed right ventricular function in 126 patients on the day of diagnosis of PE. They identified 70 patients with evidence of moderately or severely reduced right ventricular dysfunction who had nearly double the mortality rate of patients without significant right ventricular dysfunction [19]. Kasper et al. similarly found that 1-year mortality after PE was 13% in patients with evidence of right ventricular afterload stress compared with 1.3% in patients without [20]. These findings support the argument that identification of right ventricular dysfunction in patients with PE would allow for the detection of high-risk patients who could be targeted for aggressive therapy. Identification of patients by echocardiography who have right ventricular dysfunction due to PE could provide a strategy for determining who should receive aggressive reperfusion therapy.

Our own data suggest that therapy for PE is associated with recovery of right ventricular function. We studied patients with echocardiography within 48 h of PE diagnosis and on follow-up [21]. After thrombolysis, regional wall motion in 70% of right ventricular segments normalized (Fig. 6), and 15 out of 18 patients showed significant improvement in mid-free wall motion excursion. These findings suggest that recovery of right ventricular function occurs early after thrombolysis and that regional right ventricular wall motion returns to normal in the majority of patients.

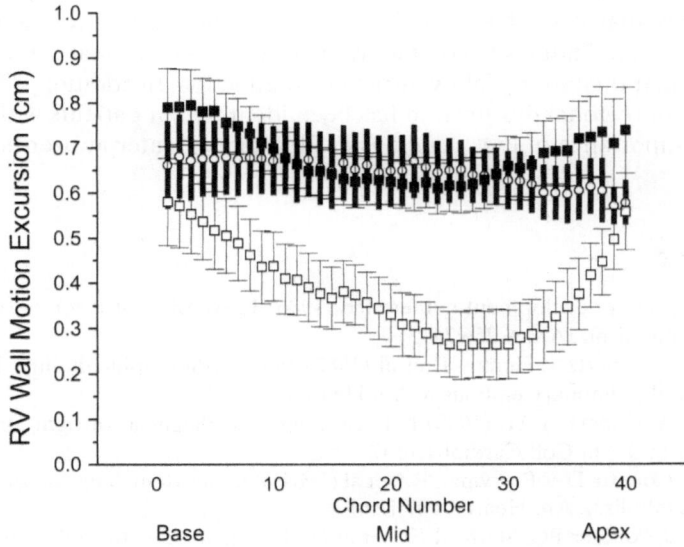

FIG. 6. Wall motion excursion (in mm) in normal controls (*open circles*; *m* = 9), patients with acute PE (*open squares*; *n* = 18), and those same patients following thrombolysis (*closed squares*; *n* = 18). Chords are displayed along the *x*-axis from the base to the apex

The Role of Echocardiography in Acute Pulmonary Embolism

Echocardiography has emerged over the past decade as an invaluable diagnostic tool in the setting of PE and one that is complementary to perfusion lung scanning and pulmonary angiography. Unlike these other commonly utilized tests, echocardiography provides functional information about the right and left ventricles that provide enormous insight into the pathophysiology and hemodynamics of the disease. Our own findings suggest that a specific pattern of regional right ventricular dysfunction can be virtually pathognomonic for PE. Nevertheless, it should be emphasized that although the specificity of this finding for PE is high, the sensitivity is not, and a normal echocardiographic examination does not exclude PE. It is likely, however, that a normal echocardiographic examination probably excludes a hemodynamically important PE. Therefore, echocardiography can and should be used as a tool to distinguish patients with hemodynamically important PE who might be targeted for aggressive therapy.

Conclusion

In summary, echocardiography provides a myriad of diagnostic information in the setting of PE. In addition to being able to visualize thrombus occasionally, echocardiography provides important functional information about the right and left ventricles that cannot be obtained by any other test. A constellation of echocardiographic findings is commonly seen in PE—abnormal septal motion, right ventricular dilatation, right ventricular dysfunction. In addition, a fairly specific pattern of regional dysfunction has been identified in patients with PE. The prognostic importance of these findings in PE makes greater awareness of them essential.

References

1. NIH Consensus development conference (1986) Prevention of thrombosis and pulmonary embolism. JAMA 256:741
2. Kasper W, Meinertz T, Henkel B et al (1986) Echocardiographic findings in patients with proved pulmonary embolism. Am Heart J 112:1284
3. Redish GA, Anderson AL (1983) Echocardiographic diagnosis of right atrial thromboembolism. J Am Coll Cardiol 1:1167
4. Percy RF, Couetta DA, Perryman RA et al (1984) Antemortem diagnosis of right atrial thromboembolism. Am Heart J 107:1278
5. Cameron J, Pohluer PG, Stafford EG et al (1985) Right heart thrombus: recognition, diagnosis and management. J Am Coll Cardiol 5:1239
6. Kasper W, Meinertz T, Kersting F et al (1980) Echocardiography in assessing acute pulmonary hypertension due to pulmonary embolism. Am J Cardiol 45:567
7. Elliot CG (1992) Pulmonary physiology during pulmonary embolism. Chest 101:163S–171S
8. McIntyre KM, Sasahara AA (1971) The hemodynamic response to pulmonary embolism in patients without prior cardiopulmonary disease. Am J Cardiol 28:288–294
9. Brooks H, Kirk ES, Vokonas PS et al (1971) Performance of the right ventricle under stress: relation to right coronary flow. J Clin Invest 50:2176–2183
10. Stein PD, Alshabkhoun S, Hawkins HF et al (1969) Right coronary blood flow in acute pulmonary embolism. Am Heart J 77:356–362
11. Mittal SR, Jain S, Maheshwari S (1996) Pulmonary embolism with isolated right ventricular infarction. Indian Heart J 48(6):704–706
12. Adams JE, Siegel BA, Goldstein JA et al (1992) Elevations of CK-MB following pulmonary embolism: a manifestation of occult right ventricular infarction. Chest 101:1203–1206
13. Kasper W, Geibel A, Tiede N et al (1993) Distinguishing between acute and subacute massive puolmonary embolism by conventional and Doppler echocardiography. Br Heart J 70:352–356
14. Feigenbaum H (1986) Echocardiography, 4th edn. Lea and Febiger, Philadelphia, p 622
15. Metz D, Chapoutot L, Ouzan et al (1991) Doppler echocardiographic assessment of the severity of acute pulmonary embolism: a correlative angiographic study in forty-eight adult patients. Am J Noninvas Cardiol 5:223–228
16. McConnel MV, Solomon SD, Rayan ME et al (1996) Regional right ventricular dysfunction detected by echocardiography in acute pulmonary embolism. Am J Cardiol 78:469–473
17. Goldhaber SZ, Haire WE, Feldstein ML et al (1993) Alteplase versus heparin in acute pulmonary embolism: randomized tiral assessing right-ventricular function and pulmonary perfusion. Lancet 341:507–511

18. Wolfe WM, Lee RT, Feldstein ML et al (1994) Prognostic significance of right ventricular hypokinesis and perfusion lung scan defects in pulmonary embolism. Am Heart J 127:1371–1375
19. Ribeiro A, Lindmarker P, Juhlin-Dannfelt A et al (1997) Echocardiography Doppler in pulmonary embolism: right ventricular dysfunction as a predictor of mortality rate. Am Heart J 134(4):479–487
20. Kasper W, Konstatinides S, Geibel A et al (1997) Prognostic signficance of right ventricular afterload stress detected by echocardiography in patients with clinically suspected pulmonary embolism. Heart 77:346–349
21. Nass N, Chyu S, Goldhaber SZ et al (1997) Recovery of regional right ventricular function after thrombolysis for pulmonary embolism. Circulation 96:1–25

Pulmonary Magnetic Resonance Angiography for Detection of Pulmonary Embolism

NORIKAZU YAMADA, HIROFUMI FUJIOKA, KIYOTSUGU SEKIOKA,
TAKAHIRO YAZU, MASHIO NAKAMURA, NAOTO HIRAOKA,
HIDEKI TANAKA, NAOKI ISAKA, and TAKESHI NAKANO

Summary. The diagnosis of pulmonary embolism may be difficult, because no reliable noninvasive imaging method is available. An accurate, noninvasive diagnostic modality is highly desirable. The purpose of this study was to evaluate the accuracy of magnetic resonance (MR) angiography in the noninvasive diagnosis of pulmonary embolism. Eighteen patients in whom the presence of pulmonary emboli was suspected underwent both conventional pulmonary angiography and MR angiography. The sensitivity and specificity of MR angiography to the level of lobar arteries were 100% and 85%, respectively, and to the level of segmental arteries, 94% and 78%, respectively. A single sectional image of MR angiography can depict thromboemboli in the proximal portion of the pulmonary arteries more definitively than conventional pulmonary angiography or a maximum-intensity-pixel projection image of MR angiography. MR angiography can reliably depict pulmonary thromboemboli down to the segmental level.

Keywords. Pulmonary embolism, Magnetic resonance angiography, Noninvasive diagnosis, Deep vein thrombosis

Introduction

The diagnosis of pulmonary embolism is still a challenge for clinicians because of its nonspecific clinical signs and symptoms, and the suboptimal accuracy of the noninvasive diagnostic modalities. Unfortunately, even the lung scan, which is the primary imaging test, is most often nondiagnostic. The lung scan is based on indirect evidence, namely the detection of perfusion abnormalities, rather than on the direct visualization of the clots themselves. The Prospective Investigation of Pulmonary Embolism Diagnosis (PIOPED) [1] clarified the diagnostic accuracy of the ventilation-perfusion scan, teaching us that a ventilation-perfusion scan with a normal or low probability of pulmonary embolism, when there is a low

The First Department of Internal Medicine, Mie University School of Medicine, 174-2 Edobashi, Tsu, Mie 514-8507, Japan

clinical suspicion, is associated with a 4% prevalence of pulmonary embolism, while a high-probability scan, coupled with high clinical suspicion, is associated with a 96% prevalence of pulmonary embolism. Although these results provide reasonable diagnostic certainty, approximately three-fourths of patients had indeterminate findings on ventilation-perfusion scan, and the presence or absence of pulmonary embolism remains uncertain. Even in patients with nondiagnostic scans, pulmonary angiography commonly reveals pulmonary embolism when the level of clinical suspicion is high. Pulmonary angiography remains the "gold standard" for accurate detection pulmonary emboli, but it is invasive, expensive, and often inconvenient. Therefore, a noninvasive and accurate diagnostic modality is highly desirable [2–5]. These approaches include D-dimer measured by enzyme-linked immunosorbent assay (ELISA), transesophageal echocardiography [6], lower-extremity ultrasonography (US) [7], spiral computed tomography (CT) [8–10], electron beam CT [11], and magnetic resonance (MR) imaging. In particular, there is currently considerable interest in the application of MR imaging techniques for the evaluation of patients suspected of having pulmonary thromboembolism. The resurgence of interest in MR for diagnosing pulmonary embolism has resulted from recent technical advances in this modality. The purpose of this study was to determine the value of this new MR angiographic technique in the diagnosis of pulmonary embolism.

Materials and Methods

Study Population

We prospectively evaluated pulmonary vascular MR angiography performed by means of SPGR (spoiled GRASS (gradient recalled acquisition in the steady state)) method in 18 patients with clinically suspected pulmonary embolism between March 1995 and April 1998. Informed consent for the MR examination was obtained from all patients.

Magnetic Resonance Angiography

All images were obtained with a standard whole-body 1.5T system (Signa, GE Medical Systems, Milwaukee, WI, USA). Typical acquisition parameters were as follows: 13.2/2.9 (repetition time (TR) ms/echo time (TE) ms); a 32 × 32-cm field of view (FOV) was used with an acquisition matrix of 256 × 128, and 5- or 10-mm-thick sections were obtained. The flip angle of the radiofrequency excitation pulse was 20°–30°. The receiver bandwidth selected by the operator was either ±16 kHz or ±32 kHz, but in most patients it was ±16 kHz. In all cases, the phased-array surface coil was used for signal excitation and reception.

A bolus of 0.1 mmol of gadolinium diethylenetriaminepentaacetic acid (Gd-DTPA) per kilogram body weight was injected manually at the highest rate possible through an 18-gauge catheter inserted in the right antecubital vein, followed by a 20-ml saline flush to ensure maximal enhancement of the pulmonary arteries. The mean duration of the injection was 15 s. Typically, patients were asked to stop breathing for 30 s.

MR angiograms were interpreted by two observers who had no knowledge of the findings on pulmonary angiography.

Pulmonary Angiography

Pulmonary angiography is considered the reference standard for diagnosis of pulmonary embolism. Accordingly, the sensitivity and specificity of MR imaging were best calculated on the basis of angiographic proof. Pulmonary angiography was performed with a 7-Fr Bermann catheter introduced into each pulmonary artery through the common femoral or internal jugular route under fluoroscopic guidance. Selective opacification of left and right pulmonary arteries was accomplished with a total dose of 75 ml of iodinated contrast material at a rate of 35 to 40 ml per injection. An intraluminal filling defect, wall irregularity, stenotic lesion, arterial web, or arterial occlusion was considered evidence of pulmonary embolism. An angiogram was considered negative whenever pulmonary embolism was not demonstrated.

Data Analysis

Correlations with findings on digital subtraction angiograms were based on the original MR report and review of the MR angiograms by two independent observers, without knowledge of the results of digital subtraction angiography.

For each MR angiographic study, the number of pulmonary arteries shown and the presence of stenosis and pulmonary emboli were determined to the level of segmental arteries. Peripheral vessels distal to segmental arteries were not estimated in this study. Partial intraluminal filling defects of abrupt vascular cutoffs with curvilinear capping of the high-signal-intensity blood column were interpreted as pulmonary emboli. No attempt was made to differentiate between acute or chronic thrombi.

Results

Eighteen patients (4 men and 14 women) with clinically suspected pulmonary embolism underwent both conventional pulmonary angiography and magnetic resonance angiography (Figs. 1–4). Their mean age was 55 years (range 38 to 77). 411 of 486 vascular segments (85%) were adequately identified by magnetic resonance angiography. The remaining 75 segments were inadequately identified because of blurring artifacts. The sensitivity, specificity, accuracy, positive predictive value, and negative predictive value of MR angiography to the level of lobar arteries were 100%, 85%, 93%, 89%, and 100%, respectively, and to the level of

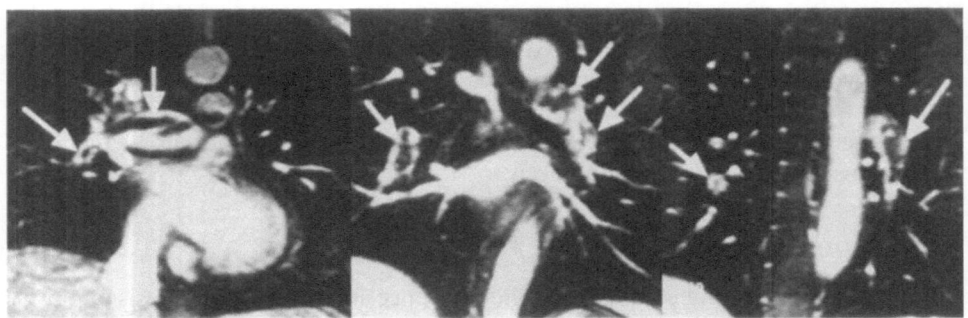

FIG. 1. Images obtained in a 59-year-old woman with syncope and dyspnea. Coronal image of magnetic resonance (MR) angiogram shows intraluminal filling defects of bilateral main and lower lobe arteries (*arrows*)

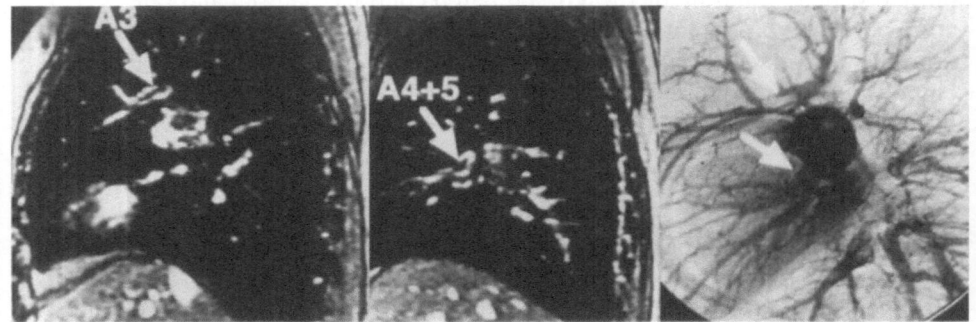

FIG. 2. *Left, middle* Sagittal image of MR angiogram shows intraluminal filling defects of right A3, A4+5 (*arrows*). *Right* Lateral view of conventional pulmonary angiogram

TABLE 1. Efficacy of pulmonary magnetic resonance (MR) angiography

	To the level of lobar arteries	To the level of segmental arteries
Sensitivity	100% (87/87)	94% (225/240)
Specificity	85% (64/75)	78% (134/171)
Accuracy	93% (151/162)	87% (359/411)
Positive predictive value	89% (87/98)	86% (225/262)
Negative predictive value	100% (64/64)	90% (134/149)

segmental arteries 94%, 78%, 87%, 86%, and 90%, respectively (Table 1). Although a maximum-intensity-pixel projection (MIP) image blurred thromboemboli in the proximal portion of the pulmonary arteries (Fig. 5), a single sectional image of MR angiogram can depict thromboemboli in the proximal portion of the pulmonary arteries more definitively than conventional pulmonary angiography.

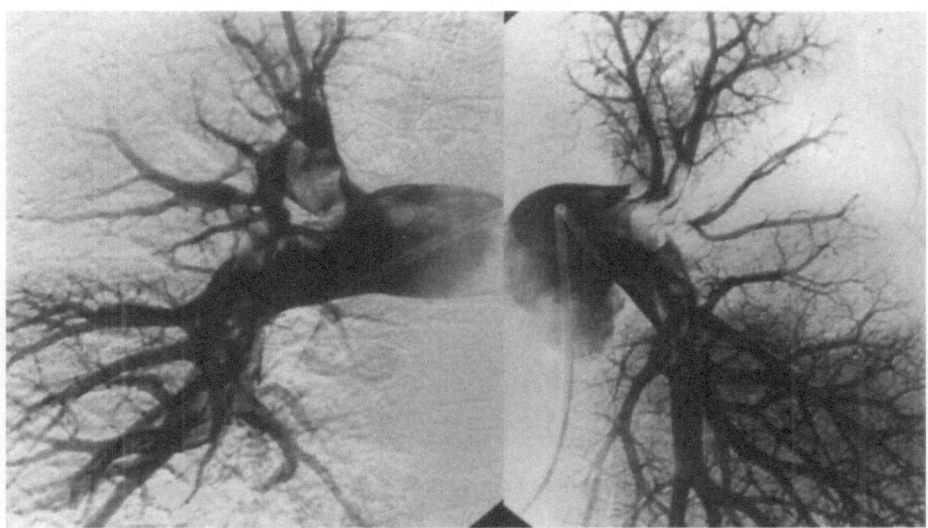

FIG. 3. Frontal views of conventional pulmonary angiogram, showing intraluminal filling defects in bilateral main, upper lobe, and lower lobe arteries. They were obtained on the same day of MR angiograms of Figs. 1 and 2

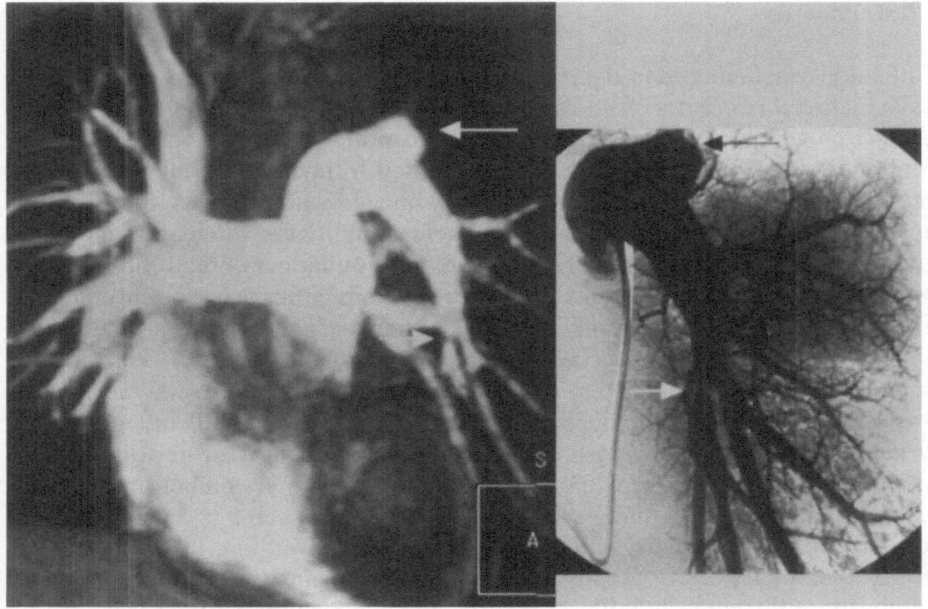

FIG. 4. Images obtained in a 66-year-old man with exertional dyspnea. *Left* coronal maximal intensity projection (MIP) image, *Right* frontal view of left conventional pulmonary angiogram, Both images can depict cutoff of left upper lobe artery and web of left A10 (*arrows*)

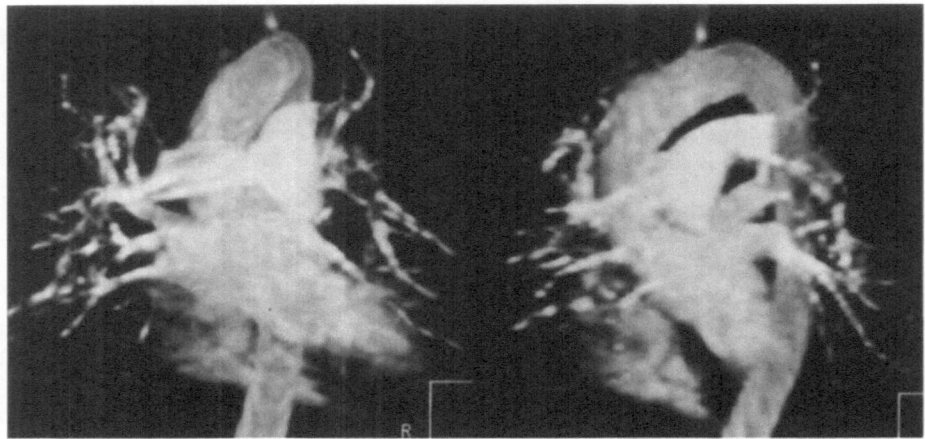

FIG. 5. MIP images in the same patient (Fig. 4). *Left* Coronal MIP. *Right* Oblique coronal MIP. MIP images blurred emboli in bilateral main pulmonary arteries compared with Fig. 1. MIP images are not suitable for the detection of proximal emboli of pulmonary arteries

Discussion

Difficulties encountered in the past with MR imaging of pulmonary vasculatures have included respiratory and cardiac motion, complicated blood-flow patterns with variable flow velocities, and magnetic susceptibility effects from adjacent air-containing lung. The initial studies were limited to imaging of only the central vessels, since peripheral vessels were poorly imaged with MR [12–16]. Recently, however, the depiction of the intraparenchymal pulmonary vasculature has been greatly improved. Schiebler et al. [17] evaluated a pulmonary breath-hold (PBH) MR angiographic technique in 18 patients in whom either acute or chronic pulmonary embolism was clinically suspected. The overall sensitivity of PBH MR angiography for detection of acute pulmonary emboli was 85%. For chronic emboli, which were smaller in anteroposterior diameter, the overall sensitivity was 42%. Diagnositic confidence greater than 75% was obtained only for emboli larger than 1 cm in anteroposterior diameter. Grist et al. [18] performed pulmonary MR angiography in 20 patients in whom pulmonary embolism was clinically suspected. They found a sensitivity of 92%–100% and a specificity of 62% for detection of pulmonary embolism. This report showed that the performance of MR pulmonary arteriography and MR venography in a single examination to demonstrate thrombus in both the arterial and deep venous systems was proved feasible.

Moreover, the development and application of macromolecular paramagnetic contrast agents that have prolonged intravascular retention, and advances in

TABLE 2. Advantages and disadvantages of pulmonary MR angiography

Advantages
No radiation exposure
No iodinated contrast material
Ability to obtain various sectional images
Ability to combine with MR venography

Disadvantages
Insufficient resolution of vessels no larger than subsegmental branches
Ghost artifact at turbulent flow
Necessity for breath holding
Inability to perform for patients with ferromagnetic object

hardware and software, such as ultrafast technique during a suspended breath, have enhanced the vascular signal intensity.

The results in our study are similar to those reported in a recent study of Meaney et al. [19]. They reported on a prospective comparison of gadolinium-enhanced magnetic resonance angiography with pulmonary angiography in 30 patients with suspected pulmonary embolism. The sensitivities were 100%, 87%, and 75%, with specificities of 95%, 100%, and 95%, respectively.

Recent technical advances in spiral and electron beam CT have also spurred a renewed interest for the noninvasive diagnosis of pulmonary embolism [20]. Remy-Jardin et al. reported results of a study to compare spiral CT with selective pulmonary angiography in 42 patients to detect central pulmonary thromboemboli. The sensitivity, specificity, and positive and negative predictive value were 100%, 95%, 96%, and 100%, respectively. The authors concluded that spiral CT can reliably depict thromboemboli in second- to fourth-division pulmonary vessels [10].

Teigen et al. reported that contrast material-enhanced electron-beam CT was performed to image the pulmonary vasculature in 86 patients. Angiographic or pathologic proof was available. The authors discovered a sensitivity of 95%, a specificity of 80%, a positive predictive value of 95%, and a negative predictive value of 80% [11].

Currently, with either MR or CT, detection of small clots in vessels at and beyond subsegmental branches is limited (see Table 2). However, it should be noted that the interreader agreement for the diagnosis of clots beyond the segmental level is low, even with conventional angiography. Furthermore, emboli in vessels no larger than subsegmental branches may not be of clinical consequence, particularly if deep vein thrombosis can be ruled out [21].

The lack of need for iodinated contrast agents and radiation and the ability to link pulmonary MR angiography with peripheral MR venography [22, 23] are additional advantages of MR imaging over CT (Fig. 6). MR angiography is

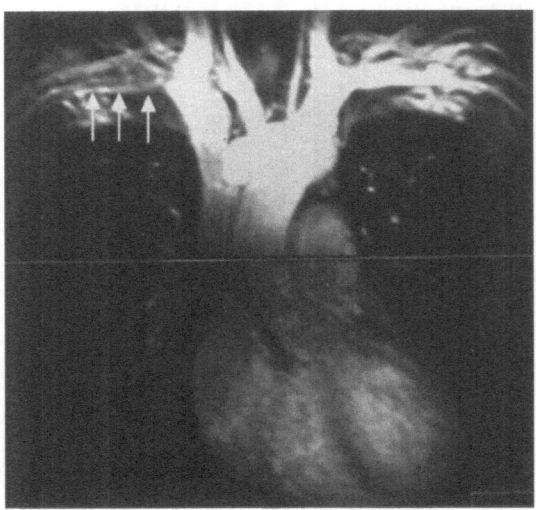

FIG. 6. MR venography used for detection of origin of emboli. Right subclavian vein is occluded (*arrows*). This 40-year-old female had massive pulmonary embolism originating in the right subclavian vein

acceptable for patients with hypersensitivity to iodinated contrast agents, since gadolinium is not nephrotoxic. In contrast, the disadvantages of pulmonary MR angiography include the necessity of breath holding, while for electron-beam CT, breath holding is not mandatory. Although supplementary oxygen enables patients with mild dyspnea to extend the duration of breath hold, MR angiography is not suitable for patients with severe hypoxemia.

MR angiography is superior to pulmonary angiography in demonstrating the mural thrombus or floating clot which occupies a small part of the vessel (Fig. 7). Whereas pulmonary angiography shows only a projection image of contrast material, MR angiography can depict various sectional images. Coronal, sagittal, axial, and oblique multiplanar images can be made available with MR angiography.

In the United States, the cost of MR imaging appears to be higher than the cost of ventilation-perfusion (V-P) scanning and CT, but lower than that of pulmonary angiography. V-P scanning is too costly to be used by itself because at least 30% of its results were nondiagnostic (low-probability and intermediate-probability scan). The implementation of a single charge of a combined MR angiographic study and MR venographic study would be comparable to the combined charges of chest CT together with a US DVT study [20]. In Japan, the cost of MR imaging is similar to that of spiral CT and lower than that of V-P scanning and angiography.

It seems probable that these new methods may obviate conventional angiography in patients with indeterminate radionuclide V-P scans and perhaps eventually may provide an alternative to V-P scanning in screening for pulmonary embolism.

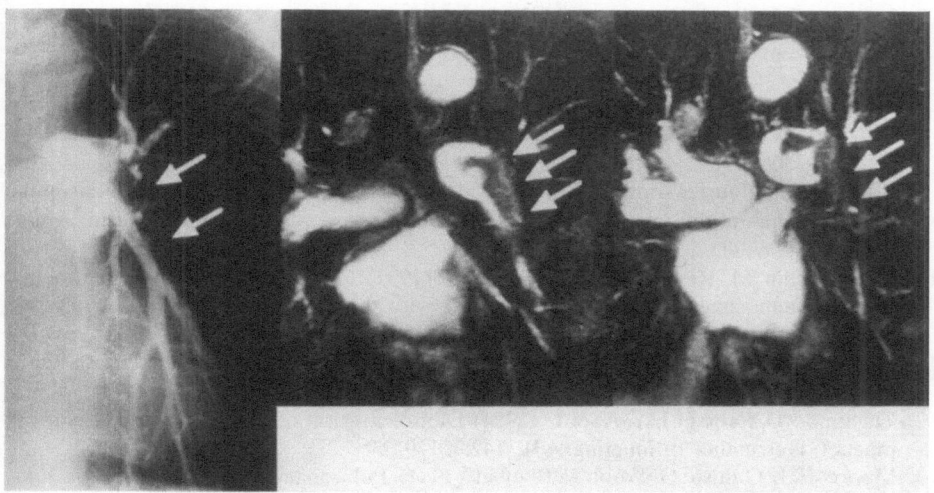

FIG. 7. Images obtained in a 67-year-old woman with chest pain and exertional dyspnea. *Left* Frontal image of conventional pulmonary angiogram of the left pulmonary artery. *Middle, right* coronal images of MR angiogram. MR angiogram shows mural thrombus in left main and lower lobe arteries more definitively than conventional pulmonary arteriogram. (*arrows*)

Conclusions

Although further advances to improve specificity of peripheral emboli are necessary, MR angiography is a promising technique for the noninvasive demonstration of pulmonary emboli and will replace V-P scanning as the screening modality for pulmonary embolism.

References

1. The PIOPED Investigators (1990) Value of the ventilation/perfusion scan in acute pulmonary embolism: results of the Prospective Investigation of Pulmonary Embolism Diagnosis (PIOPED). JAMA 263:2753–2759
2. Goodman LR, Lipchik RJ (1996) Diagnosis of acute pulmonary embolism: time for a new approach. Radiology 199:25–27
3. Tapson VF (1997) Pulmonary embolism—new diagnostic approaches. N Engl J Med 336:1449–1451
4. Fennerty T (1997) The diagnosis of pulmonary embolism. BMJ 314:425–429
5. Anderson GB (1996) Noninvasive testing in the diagnosis of pulmonary embolism. Chest 109:5–6
6. Pruszozyk P, Torbicki A, Pacho R et al (1997) Noninvasive diagnosis of suspected severe pulmonary embolism: transesophageal echocardiography vs spiral CT. Chest 112:722–728

7. Turkstra F, Kuijer PMM, van Beek EJR et al (1997) Diagnostic utility of ultrasonography of leg veins in patients suspected of having pulmonary embolism. Ann Intern Med 126:775–781
8. Remy-Jardin M, Remy J, Deschildre F et al (1996) Diagnosis of pulmonary embolism with spiral CT: comparison with pulmonary angiography and scintigraphy. Radiology 200:699–706
9. Blum AG, Delfau F, Grignon B et al (1994) Spiral-computed tomography versus pulmonary angiography in the diagnosis of acute massive pulmonary embolism. Am J Cardiol 74:96–98
10. Remy-Jardin M, Remy J, Wattinne L et al (1992) Central pulmonary thromboembolism: diagnosis with spiral volumetric CT with the single-breath-hold technique—comparison with pulmonary angiography. Radiology 185:381–387
11. Teigen CL, Maus TP, Sheedy PF et al (1993) Pulmonary embolism: diagnosis with electron-beam CT. Radiology 188:839–845
12. Thickman D, Kressel HY, Axel L (1984) Demonstration of pulmonary embolism by magnetic resonance of imaging. AJR 142:921–922
13. Moore EH, Gamsu G, Webb WR et al (1984) Pulmonary embolus: detection and follow-up using magnetic resonance. Radiology 153:471–472
14. Fisher MR, Higgins CB (1986) Central thrombi in pulmonary arterial hypertension detected by MR imaging. Radiology 158:223–236
15. White RD, Winkler ML, Higgins CB (1987) MR imaging of pulmonary arterial hypertension and pulmonary emboli. AJR 149:15–21
16. Szucs RA, Rehr RB, Tatum JL (1989) Pulmonary artery thrombus detection by magnetic resonance imaging. Chest 95:232–234
17. Schiebler ML, Holland GA, Hatabu H et al (1993) Suspected pulmonary embolism: prospective evaluation with pulmonary MR angiography. Radiology 189:125–131
18. Grist TM, Sostman HD, MacFall JR et al (1993) Pulmonary angiography with MR imaging: preliminary clinical experience. Radiology 189:523–530
19. Meaney JFM, Weg JG, Chenevert TL et al (1997) Diagnosis of pulmonary embolism with magnetic resonance angiography. N Engl J Med 336:1422–1427
20. Gefter WB, Hatabu H, Holland GA et al (1995) Pulmonary thromboembolism: recent developments in diagnosis with CT and MR imaging. Radiology 197:561–574
21. Hull RD, Rascob GE, Ginsberg JS et al (1994) A noninvasive strategy for the treatment of patients with suspected pulmonary embolism. Arch Intern Med 154:289–297
22. Bluemke DA, Wolf RL, Tani I et al (1997) Extremity veins: evaluation with fast-spin-echo MR venography. Radiology 204:562–565
23. Catalano C, Pavone P, Laghi A et al (1997) Role of MR venography in the evaluation of deep vein thrombosis. Acta Radiol 38:907–912

Management

Surgical and Transvenous Catheter Embolectomy for Acute Pulmonary Embolism: A Review

HERVÉ SORS, GUY MEYER, and PHILIPPE REYNAUD

Summary. Pulmonary embolectomy remains a treatment option for a small group of patients who have acute pulmonary embolism (PE). Surgical embolectomy under cardiopulmonary bypass (CPB) is indicated for hemodynamically compromised patients if thrombolytic treatment is contraindicated and for those with a deteriorating hemodynamic condition despite intensive medical treatment, including the use of thrombolytics. Recent reports document an average operative mortality from pulmonary embolectomy of 33% for patients undergoing pulmonary embolectomy under CPB. Numerous reports have identified an increased mortality (50%–60%) for patients who required cardiopulmonary resuscitation prior to embolectomy. In such severely compromised patients, preliminary circulatory assistance with partial femoral bypass has been advocated to allow time for diagnostic procedures, surgical preparation, induction of anesthesia, and institution of CPB. There is general agreement that embolectomy without a firm diagnostic confirmation is advocated only in exceptional cases. Although direct evidence of PE is best provided by pulmonary angiography, alternating imaging modalities (transesophageal echocardiography, spiral computed tomography angiography) may be used. The long-term prognosis is good for the majority of survivors of surgical pulmonary embolectomy. Recent transvenous embolectomy procedures have now been added to the list of management strategies. Although the role of these interventional procedures is quickly evolving, most remain poorly evaluated or even purely experimental. In institutions where the equipment and expertise for transvenous catheter embolectomy exist, this therapeutic option is an alternative if surgery is contraindicated or not readily available.

Keywords. Pulmonary embolism, Embolectomy, Transvenous catheter embolectomy

Laennec Hospital, 42 rue de Sèvres, 75007 Paris, France

Introduction

The annual incidence of venous thromboembolism in the general population of the Western world is about 1 per 1000 and that of pulmonary embolism (PE), its potentially lethal complication, 20 to 40 per 100000. Despite widespread prophylaxis in high-risk patients, acute PE remains a leading cause of morbidity and mortality, and commonly cited figures for PE-associated deaths are 100000 per year in the United States and 20000 per year in the United Kingdom [1].

While untreated PE carries a mortality rate as high as 30% [2], it has been recently shown that when correctly treated, the overall in-hospital mortality falls to below 10% and that only 0.5% to 2.5% of the patients with clinically apparent PE die from that disease [3, 4].

The hemodynamic consequences of acute embolization depend on the extent of reduction of the cross-sectional area of the pulmonary arterial bed as well as on the presence or absence of underlying cardiopulmonary disease. Although an unequivocal definition of massive PE is still lacking, a hemodynamic rather than an anatomic stratification proves to be more appropriate, the major consequence of massive PE being an increase in pulmonary vascular resistance which can result in right ventricular failure, systemic hypotension, and shock [5].

Unfortunately, very few studies of mortality in PE have been stratified according to the hemodynamic effect of the vascular obstruction. Alpert et al. reported that among 144 patients with angiographically proven PE, mortality was 5% in patients with nonmassive PE, 6% in patients with vascular obstruction greater than 50% without hypotension, and 32% in patients with massive PE and hypotension [6]. More recently, the Management Strategy and Prognosis of Pulmonary Embolism Registry (MAPPET) group reported that, among 1001 enrolled patients with massive PE and acute right ventricular failure or pulmonary hypertension, the overall in-hospital mortality rate was 8.1% in normotensive patients, 15% in patients with hypotension, 25% in shock patients, and 65% in those who required cardiopulmonary resuscitation at presentation; in all groups, death was almost always due to PE [7].

Therefore, mortality in patients without hemodynamic deterioration appears to be low, regardless of the size of the embolus, and much of the mortality in these patients stems from underlying disease rather than the impact of embolism. Conversely, the prognosis of patients with massive PE that causes hemodynamic compromise is poor under traditional care and warrants special consideration. Better therapeutic modalities, i.e., optimal antithrombotic therapy, inotropic support, and improved thrombolytic regimens [8], have led to substantial improvement and have significantly reduced the number of patients who in the past would have been considered for surgery.

Whatever the progress of PE management, the role of surgical embolectomy and of the new sophisticated transvenous procedures remains highly controversial. Part of this controversy involves the operative techniques, the lack of clinical experience for most of the catheter techniques, and the necessary preoperative diagnostic procedures; however, the major component is generated by questions regarding the indications for these procedures. The literature review reveals a wide spectrum of approaches from "no indication at all" to advocating that embolectomy should be performed in all patients in whom vascular obstruction is greater than 50% even in the absence of hemodynamic compromise [9, 10].

As will become quickly apparent in this review, a great deal of clinical judgment and experience is necessary in selecting appropriate patients for this hazardous therapy since, obviously, these patients are too rare and too ill for a randomized clinical trial. As stated by Gray et al. [11], the difficulty in defining the group of patients for whom pulmonary embolectomy is appropriate does not deny the existence of such patients, and decisions regarding surgery have (still) to be based on an individual's need.

Surgical Pulmonary Embolectomy

Historical Background

Surgery for massive PE has been a time-honored method since its first report by Friedrich Trendelenburg at the 37th annual Congress of the Deutsche Gesellschaft für Chirurgie in 1908. Unfortunately, this first operated patient died because of technical difficulties. Thereafter, Trendelenburg undertook pulmonary embolectomy on two more patients, without success. Trendelenburg himself died in 1924; in the same year, his pupil Martin Kirschner reported the first clinical success utilizing the procedure [12]. Thereafter, numerous attempts to duplicate this feat were almost universally unrewarding and, as late as 1961, only 23 reports of long-term survival after pulmonary embolectomy could be found in the world literature [13]. It was in the 1930s, while observing a patient die of massive PE, that John H. Gibbon Jr. first conceived the idea of extracorporeal circulation and, after more than two decades of investigation, first brought it to success on a human in 1954 [14].

Then, in February of 1961, Edward Sharp first used temporary cardiopulmonary bypass (CPB) for pulmonary embolectomy but did not report the case until the following year [15]. Two months latter, successful emergent pulmonary embolectomy using CPB was performed by Denton Cooley and Arthur Beall for treatment of a 37-year-old woman with acute massive PE [16]. Nearly at the same time, Allison of Oxford described a technique of bilateral embolectomy through the main pulmonary artery which used temporary venous inflow occlusion of the circulation [17].

Since that time, numerous similar successes have been reported and, although a few authors have reported a number of successful embolectomies using the venous inflow occlusion technique, the majority of surgeons now prefer the CPB technique in this procedure. The results of surgical therapy for PE were analyzed in 1967 by Cross and Mowlem [18] in a North American survey that included 137 embolectomies, 115 of which were done under CPB. Their study revealed that embolectomy carried an average 57% mortality, the range in mortality among the reporting surgeons being 0% to 100%.

Another step toward greater salvage has been the use of preoperative mechanical circulatory support to prevent death prior to embolectomy for patients who cannot immediately undergo operation. With currently available portable pump oxygenators, such patients can then benefit from preoperative cardiovascular stabilization and undergo necessary preoperative diagnostic procedures [11, 19].

Since the 1960s, the operative mortality has steadily fallen. In 1985, Del Campo reviewed 651 of the numerous reported cases of pulmonary embolectomy and calculated an overall mortality of 40% for those done with CPB [20]. These results are perhaps a little pessimistic since they include early experiences. More recent estimates of mortality in otherwise healthy patients approach 30%, a figure close to mortality with medical therapy in crudely comparable patients [21].

Operative Techniques

Three operative techniques, (1) venous inflow occlusion with normothermic cardiocirculatory arrest, (2) unilateral pulmonary embolectomy, and (3) pulmonary embolectomy under total CPB, have been used for embolectomy with minor variations [9, 22].

Inflow occlusion requires sternotomy, opening of the pericardium, and application of tapes with tourniquets around the superior and inferior venae cava in order to cross-clamp the vessels and dry out the right cardiac chambers. The pulmonary trunk is then rapidly opened and the emboli are removed. At the end of the procedure, the pulmonary artery is immediately closed with a lateral clamp and sutured after the caval tapes have been released. Periods of occlusion should be limited to 2 min with recovery periods of 15 min when repeated exploration is necessary. This method has the advantage that it can be done quickly and without special apparatus. Its disadvantages are just as obvious: there is limited time for careful exploration of the pulmonary vascular bed, and important blood loss usually occurs through the pulmonary arteriotomy. Limited experience suggests that the operative mortality of the procedure is about 60% (see below). However, the inflow occlusion technique is worth trying in the vanishingly rare situation of a patient who clearly cannot be transported to a center where CPB is available.

Unilateral pulmonary embolectomy through left or right thoracotomy is much more marginal. Although this procedure does not require apparatus for CPB, it requires more extensive preparation and therefore cannot be done as rapidly. Of more importance, the removal of emboli from the contralateral pulmonary artery is difficult. Since it is uncommon that pulmonary emboli are confined to one lung and that this situation will necessitate surgical embolectomy, the indications for this technique are still very limited.

When done with CPB, pulmonary embolectomy is a much simpler operation. In severely compromised patients, preoperative circulatory support with partial femoral bypass has been advocated to allow time for diagnostic procedures and surgical preparation until the venae cava and ascending aorta can be cannulated for complete CPB. Currently, the most commonly used procedure involves normothermic CPB with or without aortic cross-clamping. Through a lengthwise incision of the main pulmonary artery, the emboli are removed manually and by use of common bile duct forceps, standard sucking devices, or balloon catheters; the pleurae can also be opened for massaging both lungs in order to dislodge peripheral clots. The right atrium and ventricle are explored, and the inferior vena cava is flushed for residual clots. After the pulmonary trunk and the right atrium have been closed, CPB is discontinued, the cannulae are removed, and full heparinization is reversed by admistering protamine. Although CPB offers the surgeon the best conditions for embolectomy, the disadvantage of the technique is that just under an hour is required to assemble the operative team, and a broad application is still impossible because of limitation of necessary skills and facilities.

Whatever the operative procedure, the risk of subsequent fatal PE during the postoperative course is the major rationale for perioperative or postoperative inferior vena caval interruption. Although the utility of such a prophylactic maneuver makes intuitive sense, some surgeons still do not recommend systematic vena caval interruption. Direct surgical approaches (ligation and external clipping) have given way to transvenous devices introduced through the jugular or femoral vein. Since the 1980s, a number of transvenous devices have been developed (VenaTech, Bird's Nest, Titanium Greenfield, Simon-Nitinol). Long-term retrievable filters are now emerging and will probably supplant permanent filters at least in patients for whom inferior vena caval interruption is only needed for a limited time, including those who have undergone pulmonary embolectomy [23].

Results

Recent reports document operative mortality from pulmonary embolectomy that vary from one institution to another within a range of 8% to 78%, with an average mortality rate of 33% for patients undergoing pulmonary embolectomy under CPB [18, 19, 24–43] (Table 1) and 56% for those who underwent classic Trendenlenburg operation or inflow occlusion embolectomy [18,37,41,44] (Table 2). Differences in the preoperative status of patients partly explain the observed differences in survival rates from one report to another. In reviews of surgical experience, a major source of morbidity and mortality has been prolonged shock as well as preoperative cardiopulmonary arrest. Literature review clearly indicates that survival is much less likely when the patient has sustained cardiac arrest prior to embolectomy with an average survival rate as low as 43% (Table 3). In a series of 96 patients operated on at our center, multivariate analysis identified cardiac arrest and underlying cardiopulmonary disease as variables predictive of operative death that increased the mortality rate by 3.4 and 4.7, respectively [35].

Another series spanning 23 years and including 71 operated patients under CPB revealed a mortality of 11% in patients who had not suffered a preopera-

TABLE 1. Operative mortality from pulmonary embolectomy under cardiopulmonary bypass

First author [Ref.]	Publication date	No. of patients	No. of deaths	Mortality (%)
Cross [18]	1967	115	65	56
Stansel [24]	1967	10	3	30
Gentsch [25]	1969	10	3	30
Berger [26]	1973	17	4	23
Heimbecker [27]	1973	12	1	8
Reul [28]	1974	17	6	35
Tschirkov [29]	1978	24	7	29
Bottzauw [30]	1981	23	6	26
Glassford [31]	1981	20	8	40
Soyer [32]	1982	17	4	23
Mattox [19]	1982	40	22	55
Gray [33]	1988	71	21	30
Boulafendis [34]	1991	16	5	31
Meyer [35]	1991	96	36	37
Schmid [36]	1991	27	12	44
Kieny [37]	1991	122	16	13
Bauer [38]	1991	44	9	20
Meyns [39]	1992	30	6	20
Laas [40]	1993	34	15	44
Stulz [41]	1994	17	10	59
Doerge [42]	1996	36	9	25
Jakob [43]	1997	12	1	8
Total		810	269	33

[a] These figures refer to deaths that occurred intraoperatively or during the remainder of the hospitalization; reports of less than 10 cases are not included.

TABLE 2. Operative mortality from pulmonary embolectomy without cardiopulmonary bypass[a]

First author [Ref.]	Publication date	No. of patients	No. of deaths	Mortality (%)
Cross [18]	1967	11	8	73
Clarke [44]	1986	55	22	40
Kieny [37]	1991	54	42	78
Stulz [41]	1994	33	13	39
Total		153	85	56

[a] These figures refer to the classic Trendelenburg and venous inflow occlusion techniques.

tive cardiac arrest and 64% in those who had [33]. These observations are in agreement with numerous other reports that identify an increased mortality for patients who have required cardiopulmonary resuscitation prior to embolectomy [31, 36, 39, 41, 44]. In such severely compromised patients, preliminary circulatory assistance with partial femoral bypass has been advocated to allow time for diagnostic procedures, surgical preparation, induction of anesthesia, and institution of CPB [11, 19, 26, 28, 37,45].

TABLE 3. Operative mortality from pulmonary embolectomy (with or without cardiopulmonary bypass) in patients who sustain preoperative cardiac arrest

First author [Ref.]	Publication date	No. of patients	No. of deaths	Mortality (%)
Reul [28]	1974	9	4	44
Tschirkov [29]	1978	4	2	50
Glassford [31]	1981	10	5	50
Clarke [44]	1986	19	16	84
Gray [33]	1988	25	16	64
Meyer [35]	1991	24	14	58
Schmid [36]	1991	16	8	50
Kieny [37]	1991	23	11	48
Bauer [38]	1991	15	7	47
Meyns [39]	1992	12	5	50
Stulz [41]	1994	31	19	61
Doerge [42]	1996	14	8	57
Total		202	115	57

TABLE 4. Causes of operative death in 162 patients (from Refs. [19, 25–27, 29, 32, 35–37, 39, 40–42])

Cause of death	No. of deaths	Deaths (%)
Heart failure[a]	81	50
Neurological damage	32	20
Pulmonary hemorrhage	14	9
Sepsis	12	7
Diagnostic error[b]	7	4
Recurrent embolism	5	3
Miscellaneous	11	7

[a] Including right ventricular failure, left ventricular failure and cardiogenic shock of unspecified cause.
[b] No pulmonary embolism.

Operative complications are encountered often during and after surgical embolectomy. Table 4 shows the causes of the 162 operative deaths on 527 operated patients [19, 25–27, 29, 32,35–37,39–42]. Heart failure is the most frequent cause of death during pulmonary embolectomy. Other potentially lethal complications include massive pulmonary hemorrhage due to reperfusion of an ischemic or infarcted lung, adult respiratory distress syndrome, neurological damage, and postoperative mediastinitis. In a series of 96 patients, 28 out of the 60 hospital survivors (47%) experienced perioperative complications [35]. Adult respiratory distress syndrome occurred in 11 patients and bleeding in 8; 8 patients had infectious complications (2 of which were mediastinitis); other complications were neurological damage in 5 patients, acute renal failure in 5, and heparin-induced thrombocytopenia in 5.

The late prognosis is good for the majority of survivors of pulmonary embolectomy. Meyer et al. [35] reported that, during a follow-up of 56 months on average, only 6 late deaths (11%) occurred among the 55 discharged patients, and in 5 of 6 patients, death did not result from recurrent embolization or postembolic pulmonary hypertension. These observations are in line with other studies [27, 36, 39, 42, 46, 47] that did not reveal late death from recurrent or unresolved PE among patients who underwent pulmonary embolectomy. Late mortality is mainly due to comorbid conditions, particularly occult malignant disease. Furthermore, most long-term survivors have minimal residual obstruction on lung scans as well as no clinical symptoms or only mild pulmonary discomfort [46, 47]. These results indicate that in patients with a non-life-threatening disease, pulmonary embolectomy is an acceptable procedure with regard to late mortality and long-term results.

Preoperative Diagnosis

Whether a definitive diagnosis of PE is mandatory before the patient is taken to the operative room remains a point of disagreement. Although there is virtual unanimity of opinion that patients who are in a hemodynamically stable condition require an unequivocal diagnostic confirmation, this is no longer true as regards the more severely compromised patients. In such an emergency situation, many surgeons feel that if there is a high clinical suspicion of acute massive PE, then that is sufficient to undertake embolectomy [31, 36, 41, 44]. Others, however, believe that the risks of misdiagnosis are so great that every possible attempt should be made to confirm PE before an embolectomy is considered, even if this requires partial CPB while diagnostic procedures are performed [11, 19, 22, 26, 35].

Diagnostic procedures can delay surgery and consequently may contribute to mortality. Moreover, circulatory deterioration and even cardiac arrest may occur at the time of angiography [37, 41]. Although pulmonary arteriography has acquired a reputation for being a dangerous procedure in unstable patients, the risk of this procedure has now decreased markedly with improved techniques and modern low osmolar contrast media [48].

On the other hand, since mortality in patients referred for pulmonary embolectomy with an erroneous diagnosis approaches 100% [18, 44], there is general agreement that embolectomy without a firm diagnostic confirmation is advocated only in exceptional cases. Successful embolectomy also requires the presence of proximal pulmonary arterial thrombus. Distal pulmonary arterial thrombus is not accessible to the surgeon, and operation under these circumstances is almost always fatal.

Although direct evidence of PE is best provided by pulmonary angiography, alternating imaging modalities may ultimately replace pulmonary angiography, especially transesophageal echocardiography [41, 49-51] and contrast-enhanced helical CT [52], which both allow direct visualization of proximal clots. Due to the high prevalence of bilateral central thrombi in patients with hemodynamically significant PE, the diagnosis may be reliably confirmed in most cases with these techniques. As noninvasive tests with the capability of showing PE become available, these techniques may further minimize or even eliminate the diagnostic problem.

Although a high-probability lung scan is also considered as a valuable diagnostic tool, it cannot specifically diagnose proximal emboli suitable for operation and, therefore, cannot provide the sole basis for such an important therapeutic decision.

Indications

It is unlikely that a randomized trial will ever be performed comparing aggressive medical management including thrombolytic therapy to surgical therapy in massive PE. As a result, the decision whether to refer a critically compromised patient for embolectomy will continue to be highly individualized and to be guided by experience, judgment, and facilities available to the referring physician. Although the advent of thrombolytic therapy reduced the need for consideration of surgical embolectomy, contraindications to its use and refractory hypotension or shock despite optimal medical treatment have kept embolectomy a viable option unless a major comorbid illness deems it clinically inappropriate.

There is now general consensus that pulmonary embolectomy should be considered for hemodynamically compromised patients (shock) if thrombolytic treatment is contraindicated, and for those with a deteriorating hemodynamic condition despite intensive medical treatment, including the use of thrombolytics when feasible [8]. Indications for surgery also largely depend on the training and availability of the surgical team.

Transvenous Catheter Embolectomy

The concept of transvenous catheter embolectomy (TCE) was introduced in 1969 by Greenfield's group who first described the successful application of a vacuum-cup catheter device to remove experimental emboli in dogs [53]. Two years later, these authors described the successful management of acute massive PE in two patients using this new device [54]. Subsequently, the original 12 Fr double-lumen balloon-tipped catheter with a stainless-steel cup was changed to a radiopaque plastic cup with a steerable embolectomy catheter.

Since then, various other procedures and devices have been proposed for pulmonary embolectomy. Although they offer the physician a surgical alternative for the management of life-threatening PE when surgical embolectomy is not feasible, even specialized medical centers encounter such patients infrequently. In most places, TCE devices are not available on a 24-h basis, and most techniques need skill and special equipment.

Although the role of these interventional procedures is quickly evolving, most of them remain poorly evaluated or even purely experimental. Moreover, the results of catheter embolectomy have not yet improved the survival rate. As stated by Greenfield, if the concept of a catheter approach to the problem is valid, then the explanation for the failure to improve survival must relate either to the technic of its application or to the gravity of the clinical situation [55].

Clinical Experience with Greenfield's Catheter Device

The currently available device (Pulmonary Embolectomy Catheter, Meditech, Watertown, MA, USA) is a 10 Fr steerable catheter with a suction cup attached at the tip. Due to the cup's size, the catheter is inserted through the femoral or preferably the jugular vein by surgical venotomy; a steerable handle is used to control the progression of the catheter which is guided under fluoroscopy into the pulmonary artery. Clots are then removed by means of a suction cup; the procedure may have to be repeated several times in order to obtain a significant clot extraction.

To date, Greenfield's group has reported 46 patients with a 76% success rate and a 70% overall 30-day survival rate [56]. Using the same procedure in 27 patients treated from 1982 to 1994 at our institution, of whom 18 were described in 1991 [57], extraction was successful in 17 (63%) with a survival rate of 59%. Good results were associated with a shorter period from the first episode of PE (4.7 ± 5.4 days vs 18.3 ± 6.9 days) and the duration of hemodynamic impairment (13 ± 12 h vs 59 ± 38 h) [57]. Failures of the procedure were mainly associated with chronic PE resulting from multiple embolic episodes.

Catheterization of the pulmonary artery requires a skilled physician and, even with highly professional competence, the procedure is unsuccessful in 30% of the patients; these limitations may account for the infrequent use of the technique, despite impressive results in the two published series.

Clot Fragmentation by Angiographic Catheters

An alternative to Greenfield's catheter embolectomy is percutaneous catheter fragmentation and distal dispersion of proximal clots using standard angiographic catheters. Although no embolic material is removed, the dispersion of clots into the distal blood vessels will improve blood flow because of their greater vascular area relative to proximal vessels. This technique has recently gained attention because pulmonary artery catheters and guidewires are more widely available than sophisticated catheter extraction devices. Successful attempts at this simple and attractive method have been reported in 37 patients, 29 of whom have survived [58–61]; in one report, pharmacologic thrombolysis with streptokinase was combined with mechanical clot fragmentation [60]. Our experience is more disappointing since none of the six patients submitted to this procedure at our institution had clinical improvement as a result of clot fragmentation, although a significant angiographic improvement was documented in all of them.

High-Speed Rotation Catheters

Several rotational devices for mechanical thrombolysis have been introduced recently including the Kensey flexible rotating-tip catheter [62], Amplatz aspiration thrombectomy device [63], Thrombolizer device (previously Angiocor), other prototype versions of the impeller-basket catheters [64–66], and a rotatable pigtail catheter system [67]. For most of them, the fragmentation mechanism is similar: a high-speed rotation impeller is fixed within the center of a metal capsule or of a self-expandable basket which opens during rotation; the rotating inner impeller is driven by a pneumatic turbine at a speed of 100 000 to 150 000 rpm; and a strong vortex, created by the rotating device, exerts a suction effect on surrounding thrombotic material which, for some devices, is cut into fragments by the spinning basket struts.

Although most of these procedures have been successfully evaluated in vitro or in animal experiments, there are only limited clinical data. In a series of 15 patients suffering from massive PE, Dievart and associates reported the successful use of the Angiocor rotating basket catheter, resulting in a significant clinical improvement in 13 patients [68]. Results with the Amplatz thrombectomy device appear to be less satisfactory; in a series of six hemodynamically compromised patients with massive PE, pulmonary hemodynamics and clinical condition did not improve 2 h after completion of the procedure, although a 20% decrease in the angiographic vascular obstruction was observed [69].

Other Transvenous Embolectomy Procedures

Other procedures, mostly experimental, have been offered to carry out percutaneous treatment of acute venous thromboembolism, namely, high-pressure jet fragmentation and aspiration [70–72], intravascular or transcutaneous ultrasound-assisted fragmentation [73, 74], percutaneous balloon-assisted embolectomy [75], laser-assisted thrombectomy [76], and percutaneous placement of pulmonary artery metallic endoprostheses [77]. None of these methods are commonly used in clinical practice and only a few have been used to reperfuse human pulmonary arteries [72, 77].

Indications

Catheter extraction appears to be technically feasible with an acceptable mortality rate, so continued evaluation is warranted. In centers where the equipment and expertise for TCE exist, this procedure is an alternative to surgical embolectomy if surgery is contraindicated or not readily available. However, most of these procedures are not suitable for patients who have organized and adherent thrombi. Although the ease of insertion of some new TCE devices has given rise to an upward trend to widen the indications for their use, any extension of indications of TCE to other patients with massive PE warrants appropriate clinical trials. These limitations and the fact that few medical centers have gained experience in TCE may account for the infrequent use of this technique and the scarcity of published material.

References

1. Alpert JS, Dalen JE (1994) Epidemiology and natural history of venous thromboembolism. Prog Cardiovasc Dis 36:417–422
2. Barritt DW, Jordan SC (1960) Anticoagulant drugs in the treatment of pulmonary embolism: a clinical trial. Lancet 1:1309–1312
3. Carson JL, Kelley MA, Duff A et al (1992) The clinical course of pulmonary embolism. N Engl J Med 326:1240–1245
4. Douketis JD, Kearon C, Bates S, Duku EK, Ginsberg JS (1998) Risk of fatal pulmonary embolism in patients with treated venous thromboembolism. JAMA 279:458–462
5. Hoagland PM (1985) Massive pulmonary embolism. In: Goldhaber SZ (ed) Pulmonary embolism and deep venous thrombosis. Saunders, Philadelphia, pp 179–208
6. Alpert JS, Smith R, Carlson J et al (1976) Mortality in patients treated for pulmonary embolism. JAMA 236:1477–1480
7. Kasper W, Konstantinides S, Geibel A et al (1997) Management strategies and determinants of outcome in acute major pulmonary embolism: results of a multicenter registry. J Am Coll Cardiol 30:1165–1171
8. Hyers TM, Hull RD, Weg JG (1995) Antithrombotic therapy for venous thromboembolic disease. Chest 108:335S–351S
9. Meyer G, Tamisier D, Reynaud P, Sors H (1995) Acute pulmonary embolectomy. In: Goldhaber SZ (ed) Cardiopulmonary diseases and cardiac tumors, vol. III, in Braunwald E (series ed) Atlas of heart diseases. Current Medicine, Philadelphia, pp 6.1–6.12
10. Elliott CG (1995) Embolectomy, catheter extraction, or disruption of pulmonary emboli: editorial review. Curr Opin Pulm Med 1:298–302
11. Gray HH, Miller GAH, Paneth M (1988) Pulmonary embolectomy: its place in the management of pulmonary embolism. Lancet 1:1441–1445
12. Meyer JA (1990) Friedrich Trendelenburg and the surgical approach to massive pulmonary embolism. Arch Surg 125:1202–1205
13. Beall AC Jr (1991) Pulmonary embolectomy. Ann Thorac Surg 51:179
14. Gibbon JH Jr (1954) Application of a mechanical heart and lung apparatus to cardiac surgery. Minn Med 37:171–180
15. Sharp EH (1962) Pulmonary embolectomy: successful removal of a massive pulmonary embolus with support of cardiopulmonary bypass. Case report. Ann Surg 156:1–4
16. Cooley DA, Beall AC Jr, Alexander JK (1961) Acute massive pulmonary embolism. Successful surgical treatment using temporary cardiopulmonary bypass. JAMA 177:283–286
17. Allison PR, Dunhill MS, Marshall R (1960) Pulmonary embolism. Thorax 15:273–283
18. Cross FS, Mowlem A (1967) A survey of the current status of pulmonary embolectomy for massive pulmonary embolism. Circulation 35–36 (suppl 1):86–91
19. Mattox KL, Feldtman RW, Beall AC Jr, DeBakey ME (1982) Pulmonary embolectomy for acute massive pulmonary embolism. Ann Surg 195:726–731
20. Del Campo C (1985) Pulmonary embolectomy: a review. Can J Surg 28:111–113
21. Gulba DC, Schmid C, Borst HG, Lichtlen P, Dietz R, Luft FC (1994) Medical compared with surgical treatment for massive pulmonary embolism. Lancet 343:576–577

22. Sautter RD, Myers WO, Ray JF III, Wenzel FJ (1975) Pulmonary embolectomy: review and current status. Prog Cardiovasc Dis 17:371–389

23. ten Cate JW, Sors H, Goldhaber SZ (1998) Treatment of deep venous thrombosis and pulmonary embolism. In: Verstaete M, Fuster V, Topol EJ (eds) Cardiovascular thrombosis: thrombocardiology and thromboneurology. Lippincott-Raven, Philadelphia, pp 673–682

24. Stansel HC, Hume M, Glenn WWL (1967) Pulmonary embolectomy. Results in ten patients. N Engl J Med 276:717–721

25. Gentsch TO, Larsen PB, Daughtry DC, Chesney JG, Spear HC (1969) Community-wide availability of pulmonary embolectomy with cardiopulmonary bypass. Ann Thorac Surg 7:97–103

26. Berger RL (1973) Pulmonary embolectomy with preoperative circulatory support. Ann Thorac Surg 16:217–226

27. Heimbecker RO, Keon WJ, Richards KU (1973) Massive pulmonary embolism. Arch Surg 107:740–746

28. Reul GJ, Beall AC Jr (1974) Emergency pulmonary embolectomy for massive pulmonary embolism. Circulation 50 (suppl 2):236–240

29. Tschirkov A, Krause E, Elert O, Satter P (1978) Surgical management of massive pulmonary embolism. J Thorac Cardiovasc Surg 75:730–733

30. Bottzauw J, Vejlsted HJ, Albrechtsen O (1981) Pulmonary embolectomy using extracorporeal circulation. Thorac Cardiovasc Surg 29:320–322

31. Glassford DM Jr, Alford WC Jr, Burrus GR, Stoney WS, Thomas CS Jr (1981) Pulmonary embolectomy. Ann Thorac Surg 32:28–32

32. Soyer R, Brunet AP, Redonnet M, Borg JY, Hubscher C, Letac B (1982) Follow-up of surgically treated patients with massive pulmonary embolism—with reference to 12 operated patients. Thorac Cardiovasc Surg 30:103–108

33. Gray HH, Morgan JM, Paneth M, Miller GAH (1988) Pulmonary embolectomy for acute massive pulmonary embolism: an analysis of 71 cases. Br Heart J 60:196–200

34. Boulafendis D, Bastounis E, Panayiotopoulos YP, Papalambros EL (1991) Pulmonary embolism (answered and unanswered questions). Int Angiol 10:187–194

35. Meyer G, Tamisier D, Sors H et al (1991) Pulmonary embolectomy: a 20-year experience at one center. Ann Thorac Surg 51:232–236

36. Schmid C, Zietlow S, Wagner TOF, Laas J, Borst HG (1991) Fulminant pulmonary embolism: symptoms, diagnostics, operative technique, and results. Ann Thorac Surg 52:1102–1107

37. Kieny R, Charpentier A, Kieny MT (1991) What is the place of pulmonary embolectomy today? J Cardiovasc Surg 32:549–554

38. Bauer EP, Laske A, von Segesser LK, Carrel T, Turina M (1991) Early and late results after surgery for massive pulmonary embolism. Thorac Cardiovasc Surg 39:353–356

39. Meyns B, Sergeant P, Flameng W, Daenen W (1992) Surgery for massive pulmonary embolism. Acta Cardiol 47:487–493

40. Laas J, Schmid C, Albes JM, Borst HG (1993) Chirurgische aspekte zur fulminanten lungenembolie. Z Cardiol 82 (suppl 2):25–28

41. Stulz P, Schläpfer R, Feer R, Habicht J, Grädel E (1994) Decision making in the surgical treatment of massive pulmonary embolism. Eur J Cardiothorac Surg 8:188–193

42. Doerge HC, Schoendube FA, Loeser H, Walter M, Messmer BJ (1996) Pulmonary embolectomy: review of a 15-year experience and role in the age of thrombolytic therapy. Eur J Cardiothorac Surg 10:952–957

43. Jakob H, Kamler M, Vahl CF, Lange R, Tanzeem A, Hagl S (1997) Surgical alternatives in pulmonary embolism. Fibrinolysis Proteolysis 11 (suppl 2):197–203
44. Clarke DB, Abrams LD (1986) Pulmonary embolectomy: a 25 year experience. J Thorac Cardiovasc Surg 92:442–445
45. Ohteki H, Norita H, Sakai M, Narita Y (1997) Emergency pulmonary embolectomy with percutaneous cardiopulmonary bypass. Ann Thorac Surg 63:1584–1586
46. Hall RJC, Sutton GC, Kerr IH (1977) Long-term prognosis of treated acute massive pulmonary embolism. Br Heart J 39:1128–1134
47. Lund O, Nielsen TT, Ronne K, Schifter S (1987) Pulmonary embolism: long-term follow-up after treatment with full-dose heparin, streptokinase or embolectomy. Acta Med Scand 221:61–71
48. Hudson ER, Smith TP, McDermott VG et al (1996) Pulmonary angiography performed with iopamidol: complications in 1434 patients. Radiology 198:61–65
49. Deleuze PH, Saada M, de Paulis R et al (1991) Intraoperative transesophageal echocardiography for pulmonary embolectomy without cardiopulmonary bypass. Ann Thorac Surg 52:137–138
50. Torbicki A (1994) Echocardiography in pulmonary embolism. In: Morpurgo M (ed) Pulmonary embolism. Marcel Dekker, New York, pp. 153–178
51. Pruszczyk P, Torbicki A, Pacho R et al (1997) Noninvasive diagnosis of suspected severe pulmonary embolism. Transesophageal echocardiography vs spiral CT. Chest 112:722–728
52. Van Rossum AB, Pattynama PMT, Tjin A et al (1996) Pulmonary embolism: validation of spiral CT angiography in 149 patients. Radiology 201:467–470
53. Greenfield LJ, Kimmell GO, McCurdy WC (1969) Transvenous removal of pulmonary emboli by vacuum-cup catheter technique. J Surg Res 9:347–352
54. Greenfield LJ, Bruce TA, Nichols NB (1971) Transvenous pulmonary embolectomy by catheter device. Ann Surg 174:881–886
55. Greenfield LJ, Peyton MF, Brown PP, Elkins RC (1974) Transvenous management of pulmonary embolic disease. Ann Surg 180:461–467
56. Greenfield LJ, Proctor MC, Williams DM, Wakefield TW (1993) Long-term experience with transvenous catheter pulmonary embolectomy. J Vasc Surg 18:450–458
57. Timsit JF, Reynaud P, Meyer G, Sors H (1991) Pulmonary embolectomy by catheter device in massive pulmonary embolism. Chest 100:655–658
58. Brady AJB, Crake T, Oakley CM (1991) Percutaneous catheter fragmentation and distal dispersion of proximal pulmonary embolus. Lancet 338:1186–1189
59. Horstkotte D, Heintzen MP, Strauer BE, Leschke M (1991) Agressive non-surgical management of massive pulmonary embolism with cardiogenic shock. Eur Heart J 12 (suppl):52
60. Essop MR, Middlemost S, Skoularigis J, Sareli P (1992) Simultaneous mechanical clot fragmentation and pharmacologic thrombolysis in acute massive pulmonary embolism. Am J Cardiol 69:427–430
61. Heidenreich PA, Chou TM, Smedira NG et al (1995) Catheter fragmentation of massive pulmonary embolus: guidance with transesophageal echocardiography. Am Heart J 130:1306–1308
62. Stein PD, Sabbah HN, Basha MA, Popovitch J Jr, Kensey KR, Nash JE (1990) Mechanical disruption of pulmonary emboli in dogs with a flexible rotating-tip catheter (Kensey catheter). Chest 98:994–998
63. Bildsoe MC, Moradian GP, Hunter DW, Castaneda-Zuniga WR, Amplatz K (1989) Mechanical clot dissolution: new concept. Radiology 171:231–233

64. Schmitz-Rode T, Günther RW (1991) New device for percutaneous fragmentation of pulmonary emboli. Radiology 180:135–137
65. Schmitz-Rode T, Vorwerk D, Günther RW, Biesterfeld S (1993) Percutaneous fragmentation of pulmonary emboli in dogs with the impeller-basket catheter. Cardiovasc Intervent Radiol 16:239–242
66. Schmitz-Rode T, Adam G, Kilbinger M, Pfeffer J, Biesterfeld S, Günther RW (1996) Fragmentation of pulmonary emboli: in vivo experimental evaluation of two high-speed rotating catheters. Cardiovasc Intervent Radiol 19:165–169
67. Schmitz-Rode T, Günther RW, Pfeffer JG, Neuerburg JM, Geuting B, Biesterfeld S (1995) Acute massive pulmonary embolism: use of a rotatable pigtail catheter for diagnosis and fragmentation therapy. Radiology 197:157–162
68. Dievart F, Fourrier JL, Lefebvre JM et al (1994) Treatment of severe pulmonary embolism by means of a high speed rotational catheter (Angiocor Thrombolizer): first experience of mechanical thrombolysis in human beings. J Am Coll Cardiol 24:474A
69. Jagot JL, Reynaud P, Musset D et al (1997) Evaluation d'une technique de thrombolyse mécanique (thrombolyseur d'Amplatz) dans l'embolie pulmonaire massive: expérience sur patients. Rev Mal Resp 14:S30
70. Yamauchi T, Furui S, Katoh R et al (1993) Acute thrombosis of the inferior vena cava: treatment with saline-jet aspiration thrombectomy catheter. AJR 161:405–407
71. van Ommen V, van der Veen FH, Daemen MJ, Habets J, Wellens HJ (1994) In vivo evaluation of the Hydrolyser hydrodynamic thrombectomy catheter. J Vasc Intervent Radiol 5:823–826
72. Koning R, Cribier A, Gerber L et al (1997) A new treatment for severe pulmonary embolism. Percutaneous rheolytic thrombectomy. Circulation 96:2498–2500
73. Schmitz-Rode T, Günther RW, Müller-Leisse C (1991) US-assisted aspiration thrombectomy: in vitro investigations. Radiology 178:677–679
74. Bimbaum Y, Luo H, Nagai T et al (1998) Noninvasive in vivo clot dissolution without a thrombolytic drug. Recanalization of thrombosed iliofemoral arteries by transcutaneous ultrasound combined with intravenous infusion of microbubbles. Circulation 97:130–134
75. Brossmann J, Bookstein JJ (1998) Percutaneous balloon-assisted thrombectomy: preliminary in vivo results with an expandable vascular sheath system. Radiology 206:439–445
76. Meyer G, Makowski S, Steg PG et al (1991) Percutaneous pulsed dye laser recanalization of experimental venous thrombosis. Am Heart J 122:1177–1180
77. Haskal ZJ, Soulen MC, Huettl EA, Palevsky HI, Cope C (1994) Life-threatening pulmonary emboli and cor pulmonale: treatment with percutaneous pulmonary artery stent placement. Radiology 191:473–475

Clinicopathological Aspects of Chronic Pulmonary Thromboembolic Hypertension with Special Reference to Pulmonary Thromboendarterectomy in Japan

Chikao Yutani, Naoki Nishida, Masami Imakita,
Hatsue Ishibashi-Ueda, Yoshitane Tsukamoto,
Ryohei Hisaki, and Yoshihiko Ikeda

Summary. The incidence of chronic pulmonary thromboembolic hypertension (CPTEH) has been gradually increasing in Japan. Pulmonary thromboendartectomy has been recently performed, but the success rate of this operation is not as good as that in the San Diego group. To clarify the factors leading to a satistactory outcome in this operation, we have clinicopathologically compared seven autopsy cases, including three patients with CPTEH who died after operation, to 11 surgically successful patients. We have classified CPTEH to assess operative indication.

Total surgical specimens and whole pulmonary arterial trees dissected out from the proximal lobar artery to subsegmental arteries were submitted for histological examination. Serial cross sections of these specimens were made by traditional processing, cut at 5 μm in thickness, and stained with H & E, Masson trichrome, and elastica von Gieson stains. Deep vein thrombi were also sought whenever CPTEH was identified.

The results and conclusions were as follows. (1) There were minor differences in numbers and diameter, nothing less than 70%, of occluded segmental arteries between surgically successful patients and autopsy cases. The most obvious difference between them was the thickness of intima of the proximal lobar artery. In patients with surgical success, the intima of lobar arteries was thicker than that of autopsy cases. (2) The sufficient intimal thickening for successful surgery was significantly associated with a known hypercoagulable state (CPTEH-paradox?). (3) Intimal thickening of proximal lobar arteries may be required for obtaining good surgical outcome; therefore, it is of great importance to evaluate the degree of intimal thickening of the lobar artery before operation.

Department of Pathology, National Cardiovascular Center, 5-7-1 Fujishirodai, Suita, Osaka 565-8565, Japan

Keywords. Chronic pulmonary thromboembolic hypertension, Pulmonary thromboendarterectomy, hypercoagulable state, Intimal thickening of lobar artery

Introduction

Pulmonary hypertension (PH) is a pathological condition of persistent hypertension in the pulmonary circulation system. An important criterion in its diagnosis is an average resting pulmonary artery systolic pressure of over 30 mmHg [1]. Pulmonary hypertension is known to occur in many diseases, such as congenital and valvular heart diseases [2]. On the other hand, there exists a group of pulmonary hypertension in which there is no definite cause, or there is an underlying disease, but the mechanisms by which PH develops remain unknown. These include idiopathic pulmonary hypertension which is synonymous with primary pulmonary hypertension, pulmonary hypertension occurring in various collagen vascular diseases [3, 4], and pulmonary hypertension associated with hypercoagulable states such as protein C deficiency or the lupus anticoagulant (LA) syndrome [5, 6].

We have experienced 18 candidate patients who had chronic pulmonary thromboembolic hypertension (CPTEH) associated with protein C deficiency, LA-positive and collagen disease such as systemic lupus erythematosus (SLE), and mixed connective tissue disease (MCTD) [7]. The incidence of CPTEH in Japan has been increasing. Although pulmonary thromboendarterectomy has been recently performed [8], the success rate of this operation is not as good as that of the San Diego group [9, 10]. To explore the factors leading to success, we have clinicopathologically compared autopsy cases of surgically failed patients with CPTEH to surgically successful cases. We have classified CPTEH for the purpose of the assessment of operative indication.

Materials and Methods

The autopsy and surgical records of all patients with established diagnosis of CPTEH, who died or underwent thromboendarterectomy in the National Cardiovascular Center from 1977 to 1998, were investigated.

There were 14 surgical cases of CPTEH, including 3 patients who died after operation. There were four autopsy cases of CPTEH, candidates for operation who never underwent surgery. All autopsy cases having CPTEH as a significant cause of death were further evaluated and the clinical data from the autopsy records were analyzed.

Pathological examinations were done as follows.

Surgical Cases. After taking photographs at the time of thromboendarterectomy, total surgical specimens were submitted for histological examination. Serial cross-sectioning of these specimens was made by traditional processing, cut at

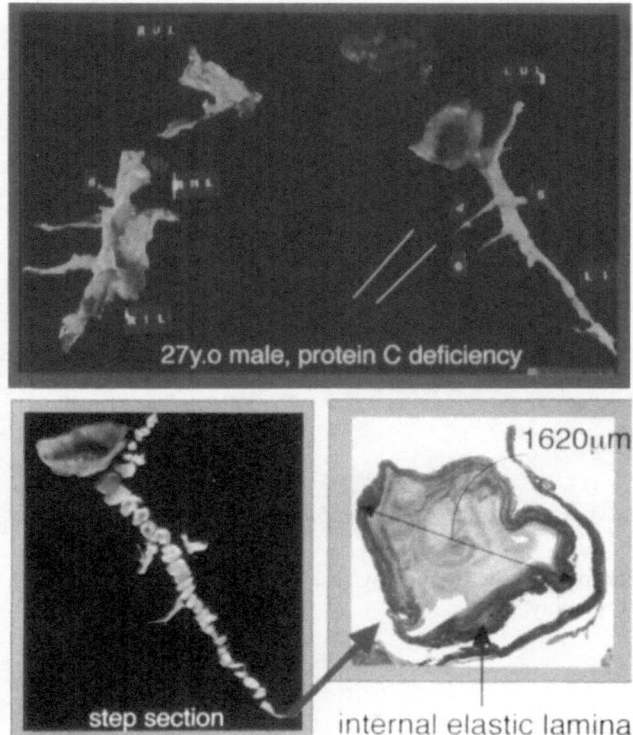

FIG. 1. Gross microphotographs of a surgically successful patient with pulmonary thromboendarterectomy. The diameter of the most distal accessible lesions was mainly 1500–2000 μm, which was consistent with segmental to orifice of subsegmental arteries

5 μm in thickness, and stained with H & E, Masson trichrome, and elastica von Gieson stains (Fig. 1).

Autopsy Cases. After documenting of the weight of lungs, location of infarcts, and postmortem pulmonary angiography data, we dissected out whole pulmonary arterial trees from the proximal lobar artery to subsegmental arteries, and performed the same methods as with the surgical specimens mentioned above. Deep vein thrombi were sought whenever CPTEH was identified. The inferior vena cava, external iliac veins, and the deep pelvic veins were examined. The proximal femoral veins were also exposed (Fig. 2) [11, 12].

We carried out morphometric measurements and analysis using a light microscope equipped with a micrometer, and measured the thickness of the intima, i.e., from the internal elastic laminae to the epithelium of the most thickened intima, and the diameter, i.e., the distance between the internal elastic laminae.

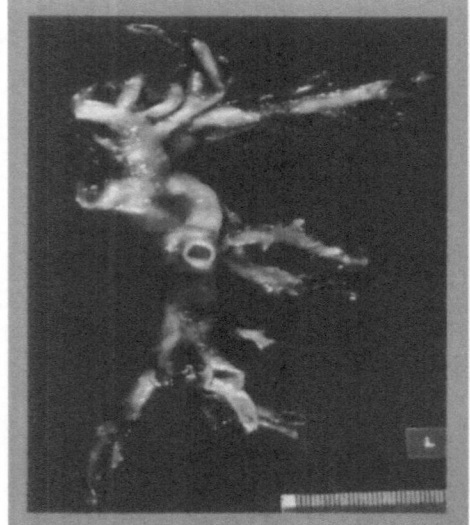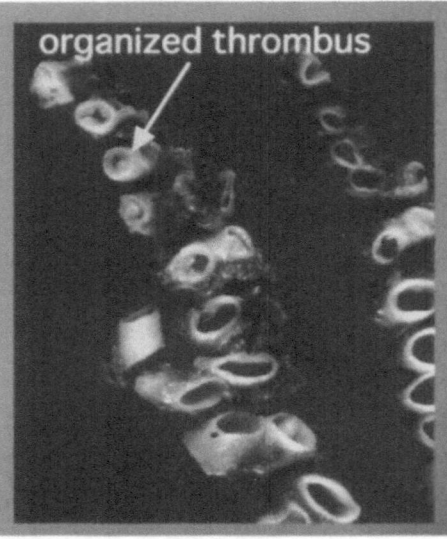

FIG. 2. Gross photographs of an autopsy case who died after pulmonary thromboendarterectomy

Results

Clinical Features

The mean age of 11 patients on whom PTE was successfully performed was 39.7 years. Seven were male and four were female. The mean age of male patients was 34.5 years, and of female patients 48.8 years. Preoperative hemodynamic data disclosed that the mean pulmonary artery pressure was 45.2 mmHg, and the calculated pulmonary vascular resistance was 15.6 mmHg/l per minute (Table 1).

Postoperatively, in patients in whom valid postoperative hemodynamic values were available, highly significant ($P < 0.001$) decreases occurred in both mean pulmonary artery pressure (45.2 to 13.8 mmHg) and pulmonary vascular resistance (15.6 to 3.4 mmHg/l per minute). (Table 1).

Hypercoagulable states such as protein C deficiency, AT-III deficiency, and positive lupus anticoagulant was found in 7 surgically successful patients, and in 1 of 7 surgically unsuccessful and inoperative autopsy patients (Table 2).

Pathology Results

We conducted morphometry on pulmonary arteries, in which the most distal occlusions of the organized thromboemboli were seen, from the tissue blocks of these two groups. In both groups, the most distal portion of thromboemboli

TABLE 1. Clinical outcome

	Successful cases (n = 11)	Autopsy cases (n = 7)
Male (average age)	n = 7 (34.5 y.o.)	n = 1 (64 y.o.)
Female (average age)	n = 4 (48.8 y.o.)	n = 6 (56.8 y.o.)
Total (average age)	39.7 y.o.	57.8 y.o.
mPA (mmHg)		
Preoperative	45.2	51.0
Postoperative	15.6	ND
TPR (mmHg/l/min)		
Preoperative	13.8	ND
Postoperative	3.4	ND

y.o., years old; mPA, mean pulmonary artery pressure; TPR, total pulmonary vascular resistance; ND, not determined.

TABLE 2. Pathological data

	Surgical cases (successful) (n = 11)	Autopsy cases (unsuccessful or inoperative) (n = 7)
DVT	9/11	4/7
Abnormal blood coagulation[a]	7/11	0/7
	$P < 0.02$	
Intimal thickness of lobar artery	>400 μm	<400 μm
Diameter of most distal occuluded artery		
>1500–2000 μm	100%	70%–90%
<1500 μm		10%–30%

DVT, deep vein thrombosis. [a] Protein C deficiency (1), protein C, S deficiency (1) antithrombin III deficiency (1), antiphospholipid syndrome (4).

lodged in pulmonary arteries was approximately 1500 μm in diameter, and more than 70% of segmental and/or subsegmental arteries were occluded by organized thromboemboli. Surgically failed and inoperative autopsy cases, however, showed that the intima of lobar arteries was less than 400 μm in thickness, which appeared to be normal intima. On the contrary, surgically successful patients had more than three times the normal intimal thickness. As for deep vein thrombosis (DVT), the surgically successful group showed DVT clinicopathologically in 7 of 11 patients, whereas the surgically failed and autopsy group showed DVT in 3 of 7 patients (Table 2).

Discussion

We performed the same operative procedure for CPTEH in the National Cardiovascular Center as described by Jamieson et al. of the University of California at San Diego [10]. Compared with their much better experience, it should be said that our experience is undoubtedly premature because of the low number of patients and our "learning curve". Moreover, the number of the patients who had pulmonary thromboendarterectomy was not only very small, but also our results might reflect only one aspect of this operation. Surgical outcome obtained in our center was not as good that obtained by Jamieson et al.; therefore, we explored the factors influencing the poor outcome. Our results revealed the following. (1) There were minor differences in numbers and diameter, nothing less than 70%, of occluded segmental arteries between surgically successful patients and autopsy cases. The most obvious difference between them was the thickness of intima of the proximal lobar artery. In patients with surgical succeess, the intima of lobar arteries was thicker than that of autopsy cases. (2) The sufficient intimal thickening for successful surgery was significantly associated with a known hypercoagulable state (CPTEH-paradox?). (3) Intimal thickening of proximal lobar arteries may be required for obtaining good surgical outcome; therefore, it is of great importance to evaluate the degree of intimal thickening of the lobar artery before operation.

Generally speaking, hypercoagulable states such as protein C deficiency, AT-III deficiency, and positive lupus anticoagulant were thrombogenic in artery and vein, so a high prevalence of deep vein thrombosis in this particular series i.e., the surgically successful case group, is more likely to have thickened intima [3–7].

A vital aspect of this pulmonary thromboendarterectomy program has been the presence of an experienced and highly interactive medical-surgical team for the preoperative evaluation of, surgical approach to, and postoperative management of patients with this complex condition [9]. The ability to safely perform good quality pulmonary angiograms and to perform angioscopy in cases of doubt are fundamental to success, as seen in our surgically failed patient group. Safe and expeditious placement filters in the inferior vena cava and careful anticoagulant management, including meeting the challenge of coagulopathies such as heparin-associated thrombocytopenia, are all important elements in reducing mortality and morbidity and in achieving satisfactory long-term outcomes [9].

From the pathological viewpoint, however, the most critical finding was whether the thickness of the lobar arteries is sufficient for continuous access until organized thromboemboli could be lodged in segmental artery and/or subsegmental artery.

Christman and colleagues [13] have shown that patients with primary pulmonary hypertension have an abnormally elevated ratio of the metabolites of thromboxane and prostacycline; since thromboxane is a potent pulmonary vasoconstrictor and promotes platelet aggregation whereas prostancyclin has the opposite effects, this imbalance could contribute to both pulmonary vasoconstriction and local thrombosis.

To describe in more detail the surgical outcome of pulmonary thromboendaterectomy in our center, we need to acquire further experience of this operation in future.

References

1. Rubin LJ (1997): Primary pulmonary hypertension. N Engl J Med 336:111–117
2. Wagenvoort CA, Mooi WJ (1989) Biopsy pathology of the pulmonary vasculature. Chapman and Hall, London, pp 128–148
3. Kusukawa R, Nishimaki T, Takagi T et al (1990) Pulmonary hypertension in connective tissue disease—clinical analysis of sixty patients in a multiinstitutional study. Clin Rheumatol 9:56
4. Miyata M, Kida S, Kanno T et al (1992) Pulmonary hypertension in MCTD: report of two cases with anticardiolipin antibody. Clin Rheumatol 11:195
5. Asherson RA, Mackworth-Young CG, Boey ML et al (1983) Pulmonary hypertension in systemic lupus erythematosus. Br Med J 287:1024
6. Clerk LSD, Michielsen PP, Ramael MR et al (1991) Portal and pulmonary vessel thrombosis associated with systemic lupus erythematosus and anticardiolipin antibodies. J Rheumatol 18:1919
7. Yutani C, Imakita M, Ishibashi-Ueda H et al (1995) Pulmonary thromboembolic hypertension in systemic lupus erythematosus with lupus anticoagulant: histopathological analysis of localization and distribution of thromboemboli in pulmonary vasculature. Intern Med 34:1030–3034
8. Okubo S, Naito M, Fukunaga Y et al (1983) Recurrent pulmonary embolism. Jpn Circ J 47:543–551
9. Mosar KM, Bloor CM (1993) Pulmonary vascular lesions occurring in patients with chronic major vessel thromboembolic pulmonary hypertension. Chest 103:685–692
10. Jamieson SW, Auger WR, Fedullo PE et al (1993) Experience and results with 150 pulmonary thromboendarterectomy operations over a 29-month period. J Thorac Cardiovasc Surg 106:116–127
11. Morpurgo M, Schmid C (1995) The spectrum of pulmonary embolism, clinicopathologic correlations. Chest 107:18S–20S
12. Chau KY, Uuen ST, Wong MP (1997) Clinicopathological pattern of pulmonary thromboembolism in Chinese autopsy patients: comparison with caucasian series. Pathology 29:263–266
13. Christman BW, McPherson CD, Newman JH et al (1992) An imbalance between the excretion of thromboxane and prostacyclin metabolites in pulmonary hypertension. N Engl J Med 327:70–75

Emergent Pulmonary Embolectomy: The Efficacy of Percutaneous Cardiopulmonary Support as a Bridge to Surgery

HITOSHI OHTEKI[1], KOJIRO FURUKAWA[1], HIROYUKI OHNISHI[1], YASUSHI NARITA[1], TSUYOSHI ITO[2], and SATOSHI OHTSUBO[2]

Summary. Five patients with acute pulmonary embolism (APE) underwent operation by the author between 1985 and 1990 because of circulatory collapse. All were weaned from extracorporeal circulation, but two patients were lost because of bleeding tendency and neurological deficit. Considering such experiences until 1990, we have changed our strategy in the surgical management of APE at our institution. Since 1991, 33 patients with massive APE have been treated, most with thrombolytic therapy. Transthoratic echocardiogram is very effective in detecting APE as an initial diagnostic procedure and confirmed marked dilation of the right ventricle with a small left ventricle. Four patients were seen with severe cardiopulmonary collapse, and all received cardiopulmonary resuscitation. Acute pulmonary embolism was strongly suspected, and percutaneous cardiopulmonary support (PCPS) was initiated for resuscitation and the maintenance of circulation for three patients. After resuscitation, transesophageal echocardiography was done and showed thrombus in the main pulmonary artery. Three patients were taken to the operating room without the conventional definitive diagnostic studies. One patient responded to resuscitation without PCPS, underwent pulmonary angiography, and received thrombolytic therapy followed by emergent pulmonary embolectomy. All four patients were subsequently discharged from the hospital and are doing well now. The clinical course of the four patients is described, and management of massive pulmonary embolism and the efficacy of PCPS as a bridge to operation are discussed. It is concluded that surgical treatment for moribund APE is effective and can be performed safely, and PCPS is also effective as a bridge to operation or alternative diagnostic procedure or treatment.

[1] Department of Cardiovascular Surgery, Saga Prefectural Hospital Koseikan, 1-12-9 Mizukae, Saga 840-8571, Japan
[2] Department of Thoracic and Cardiovascular Surgery, Saga School of Medicine, 5-1-1 Nabesima, Saga, Japan

Keywords. Acute pulmonary embolism, Emergent pulmonary embolectomy, Percutaneous cardiopulmonary support, Transesophageal echocardiogram

Introduction

The incidence of acute pulmonary embolism (APE) in Japan has been low in comparison with that in the United States and Europe [1]. Although the estimate for embolism in all actuality is underestimated, it is likely that prevalence of the disease is increasing in Japan, probably due to an increase in the modern Japanese life style. As treatment, conservative anticoagulation is effective for most patients [2, 3]. In the remaining patients, anticoagulation alone is insufficient. Some of these patients are candidates for thrombolytic therapy. For a few, however, pulmonary embolectomy may represent the only chance for survival [4, 5]. This paper reviews our experiences with surgical treatment and strategy for APE and discusses the role of percutaneous cardiopulmonary support (PCPS) as a bridge to pulmonary embolectomy.

Materials and Methods

From April 1985 to December 1990, the author operated on five patients for APE in another hospital at the request of cardiologists (Table 1, patients 1–5). There were two men and three women, aged 36 to 81 years. The diagnosis of the patient 1 was initially thought to be acute myocardial infarction and percutaneous transluminal coronary angioplasty was scheduled, but turned out to be acute massive pulmonary embolism. Thrombolytic therapy was originally chosen for him considering his old age, but eventually he required surgery because of the unstable hemodynamics. Hypotension and hypoxemia were caused by acute pulmonary embolism in patient 2 after receiving radiation therapy for uterine cancer. Although thrombolysis was performed, her hemodynamic status worsened with catecholamines. Patients 3 and 4 underwent neurologic surgery and developed cardiac arrest on postoperative days 2 and 7, respectively. Patient 5 suffered hypotension due to APE without any underlying disease. The lessons we learned from these cases were the need for early diagnosis and optimal and effective thrombolytic therapy. Also, we became aware of the potential risk of embolism after neurologic surgery. These experiences motivated us to devise a management strategy for acute pulmonary embolism.

From January 1991 to December 1997, we have managed 33 patients with acute pulmonary embolism. Most were treated successfully with thrombolytic therapy. There were 16 women and 17 men, aged 39 to 94 years with a mean age of 69 years. Four patients underwent emergent pulmonary embolectomy (Table 1, patients 6–9). There were two men and two women, aged 37 to 76 years. Patients 6, 8, and 9 were recovering from surgical procedures, and patient 7 had been

TABLE 1. Surgical cases of acute pulmonary embolism

1. Male, 81 years:
   chest pain → AMI → APE → UK 1 000 000 U → hypoxemia, hypotension → surgery
   → bleeding tendency → died
2. Female, 36 years:
   uterine cancer op and radiation, dyspnea, hypoxemia → admit and UK → hypoxemia,
   hypotension → surgery → alive
3. Female, 48 years:
   neurosurgery postop 2 days → sitting position → chest pain, dyspnea → UK → hypoxemia,
   hypotension → cardiac arrest → surgery → died
4. Female, 49 years:
   neurosurg postop 7 days → chest pain, dyspnea → cardiac arrest → surgery → alive
5. Male, 49 years:
   chest pain, dyspnea → admit and UK → hypoxemia, hypotension → surgery → alive
6. Male, 72 years:
   post uro op → bedside standing → dyspnea → cardiac arrest → no response to CPR → PCPS
   → alive
7. Female, 53 years:
   bed rest → 1st sitting position → dyspnea → cardiac arrest → no response to CPR → PCPS
   → alive
8. Female, 76 years:
   post uro op → bedside standing dyspnea → cardiac arrest → no response to CPR → PCPS
   → alive
9. Male, 37 years:
   post ortho op → 1st sitting position → dyspnea, chest pain, shock → CPR → thrombolysis
   → CRBBB, af, hypotension → alive

Patients 1–5 underwent emergency pulmonary embolectomy at other institutions, and patients 6–9
underwent the same procedure at our hospital (Saga Prefectural Hospital).
AMI, acute myocardial infarction; APE, acute pulmonary embolism; UK, Urokinase; CPR cardiopulmonary resuscitation; PCPS, percutaneous cardiopulmonary support; CRBBB, complete right
bundle branch block; af, atrial fibrillation.

treated as unknown origin lower limb paralysis. All suffered acute cardiopulmonary collapse and remained hypotensive and hypoxic despite intravenous
fluids, vasopressors, and 100% inspired oxygen. Transthoracic echocardiography
(TTE) demonstrated marked dilation of right ventircle and a small left ventricle.
Finally, all patients required temporary external cardiac massage. Acute pulmonary embolism was strongly suspected. Percutaneous cardiopulmonary
support (PCPS) was initiated for the resuscitation and maintenance of circulation in 3 patients (patients 6, 7, and 8). For arterial cannulation, the short 16 Fr
cannula was used, and the long 20 Fr cannula was used for venous cannulation.
After introduction of PCPS, two of the three patients regained consciousness.
One patient responded to resuscitation without PCPS (patient 9). After resuscitation, Transesophageal echocardiography (TEE) was done and showed thrombus in the main pulmonary artery in all.

Pulmonary arteriography was done in patient 9 for definitive diagnosis, and
although selective intrapulmonary artery thrombolysis therapy was performed,
profound hypotension persisted.

The operative technique was uniform for each patient; access was by median sternotomy. After cannulation of the aorta and vena cava, the patients were placed on cardiopulmonary bypass. Thrombi were extracted through the main pulmonary arteriotomy and right main pulmonary arteriotomy between superior vena cava and aorta. The pleural space was not opened and peripheral clots were extracted through the arteriotomy with a soft suction tube. Clipping of the inferior vena cava was not performed. Representative thrombi extracted from patient 9 are shown in Fig. 1.

Results

From April 1985 to December 1990, all patients were weaned from extracorporeal circulation. Patient 1 died because of liver failure caused by massive transfusion and bleeding due to shock, thrombolytic therapy, and extracorporeal circulation. Patient 3 died of neurological deficit 2 days after neurological operation. Patient 5 died 3 years after the operation because of uterine cancer. The other 2 patients are doing well now.

From January 1991 to December 1997, all patients improved postoperatively and were weaned from vasopressors and mechanical ventilation. Sodium warfarin was started on the second postoperative day. All patients had a lung scan at 3 months after discharge, which showed no perfusion defects. All patients are doing well now.

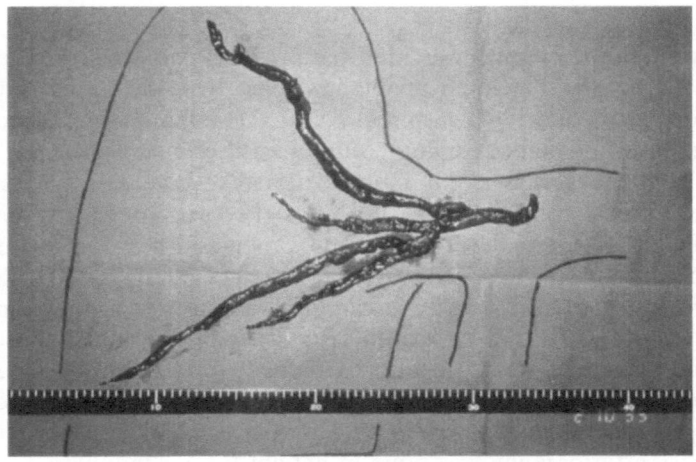

Fig. 1. Representative thrombi extracted from patient 9. The thrombus shows the shape of the pulmonary artery tree

Discussion

Massive pulmonary embolus usually leads to in-hospital death if not treated aggressively. Goldhaber [2] pointed out 12 clinical signs of acute right ventricular failure that were suggestive of a pulmonary embolism. These signs may not be present, and if present they may be misleading to date. It has been estimated that APE are increasing in number in Japan and are responsible for factors of in-hospital death [6]. The estimate for embolism in all actuality is probably low compared with Western countries, and diagnostic strategy is not well established in Japan [1]. We have now devised our strategy for diagnosis and management of APE (Fig. 2). In some instances, however, the degree of compromise is so severe that an immediate move to the operating room is indicated. In such circumstances, TEE is very effective for the diagnosis for pulmonary embolism, and thrombus may be seen in the main pulmonary artery in some cases (Fig. 3). We performed TEE in massive pulmonary embolism in 8 cases and thrombus could be seen 7 of these cases. Computed tomography scanning gives us information about thrombus in the pulmonary arteries and also provides additional information concerning pathology of the lung, heart, and great vessels (Fig. 4).

Meyer and associates [7] reported that the mortality rate of emergency pulmonary embolectomy for patients after a preoperative cardiogenic arrest was high as 58%. Mattox and associates [8] reported a salvage rate of 50% for the moribund patients and first reported the assocition of surgically introduced partial cardiopulmonary bypass for critically ill patients.

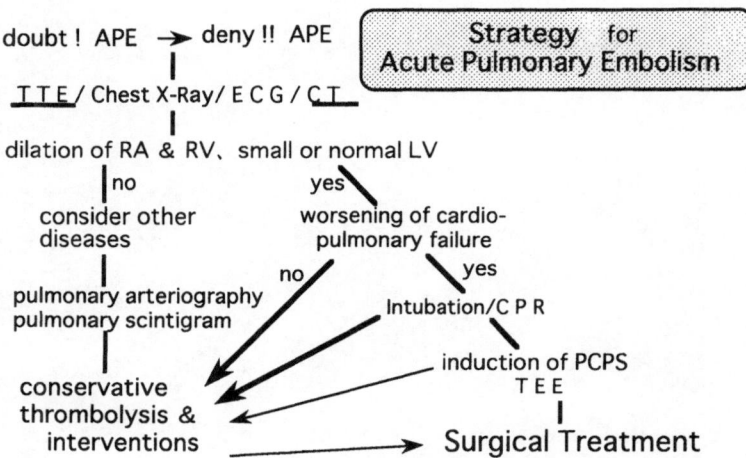

FIG. 2. Current strategy for acute pulmonary embolism (*APE*). *TTE*, transthoracic echocardiography; *CT*, computed tomography; *RA*, right atrium; *RV*, right ventricle; *LV*, left ventricle; *CPR*, cardiopulmonary resuscitation; *PCPS*, percutaneous cardiopulmonary support; *TEE*, transesophageal echocardiography

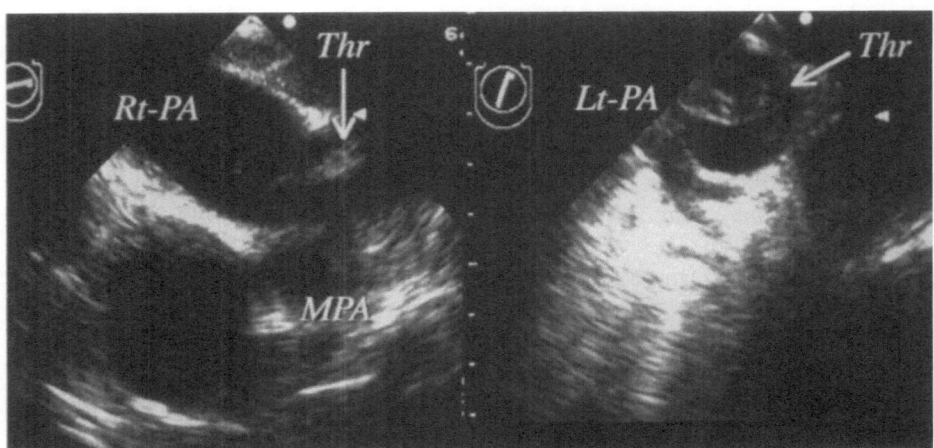

FIG. 3. Representative case of transesophageal echocardiography detected thromboem-bolus (*Thr*) in the main pulmonary artery (*MPA*). *Rt*, right; *Lt*, left

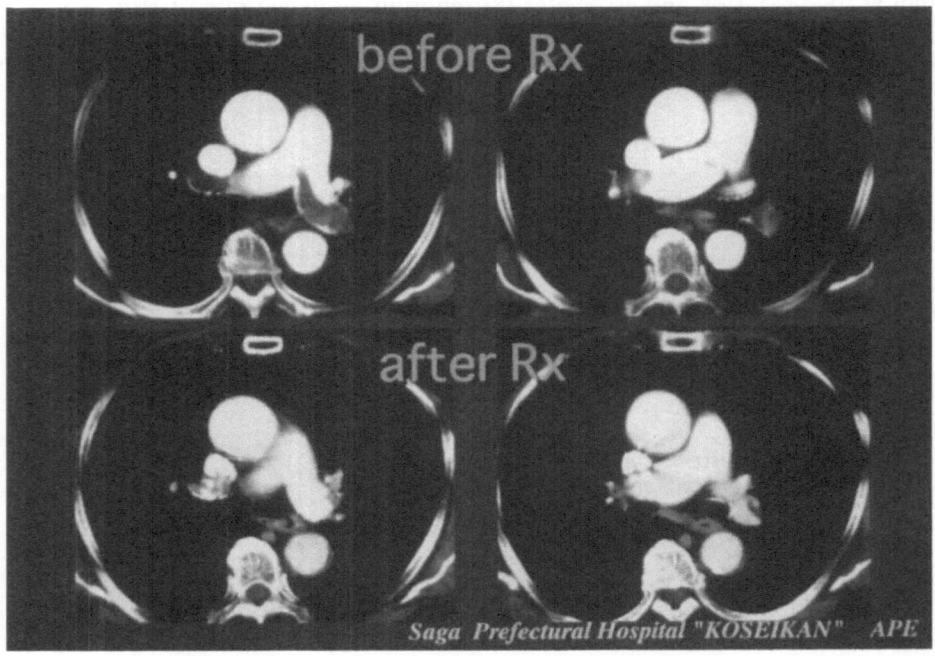

FIG. 4. Thrombus detected with computed tomography scan before thrombolytic therapy and dissolved after treatment

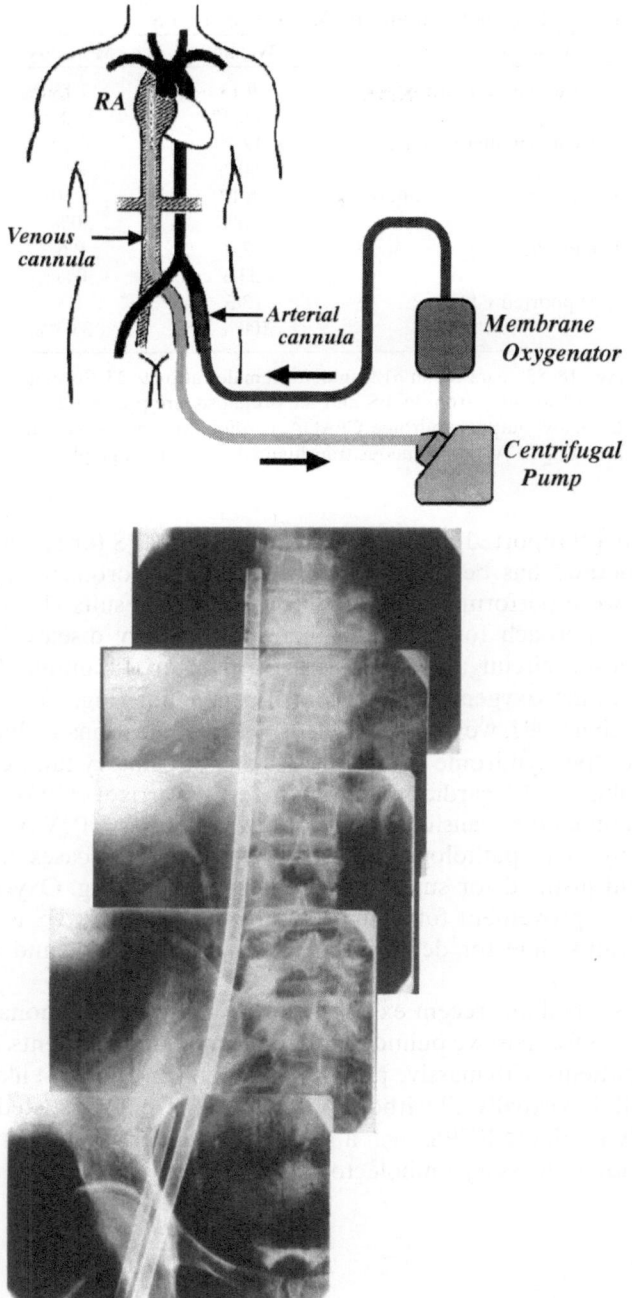

FIG. 5. Schematic drawing of percutaneous cardiopulmonary support (*top*) and real imaging of the cannula (*bottom*)

124   H. Ohteki et al.

Table 2. Indication among 52 cases of PCPS

Classification	Weaned	Mortality
1. Postcardiotomy LOS	9/13	7/13
	69.2%	53.8%
2. Acute circulatory failure	12/20	6/20
	60%	30%
3. Acute respiratory failure	6/10	5/10
	60%	50%
4. CPAOA	2/6	0/6
	33.3%	0%
5. Supported PTCA	3/3	1/3
	100%	33.3%

Age 18–83 years, mean 61.9; male to female ratio 29:23. Success rate of weaning from PCPS, and the prognosis, are presented. LOS, low output syndrome CPAOA, cardiopulmonary arrest on arrival; PTCA, percutaneous transluminal coronary angioplasty.

Phillips et al. [9] reported the initial experience of PCPS for refractory cardiac arrest. This method has been widely developed, and coronary angioplasty or valvuloplasty were performed using PCPS with good results [10, 11]. We have also used this approach for refractory cardiorespiratory disease [12–14]. This system is a closed circuit and includes a short arterial cannula, long venous cannula, membrane oxygenator, and centrifugal pump (Fig. 5). From January 1991 to December 1997, we had 52 cases of PCPS. Indications included postcardiotomy low output syndrome (LOS) in 13, acute circulatory failure in 20, acute respiratory failure in 10, cardiopulmonary arrest on arrival (CPAOA) in 6, and support of percutaneous transluminar coronary angioplasty (PTCA) in 3. Success varies according to the pathology of the patient (Table 2). In cases of APE, PCPS is effective and justified for support of both heart and lung. Oxygenation and hemodynamic improvement following the introduction of PCPS is usually dramatic and permits time for definitive diagnosis, if necessary, and transport to operation.

We have described our recent experience with emergent pulmonary embolectomy using PCPS for massive pulmonary embolism in three patients. In the group of moribund patients with massive pulmonary embolism, the most likely outcome would be death in virtually all without operation or strongly assisted circulation. With currently available PCPS, such a patient can undergo emergent diagnostic procedures and, if recessary, embolectomy.

References

1. Mieno T, Kitamura S (1989) Pulmonary thrombo-embolism—the real state in Japan in Japanese with English translation. Kokyu to Junkan 37:923–927
2. Goldhaber SZ (1991) Thrombolysis for pulmonary embolism. Prog Cardiovasc Dis 34:113–134

 3. Konstantinides S, Geibel A, Olschewski M et al (1997) Association between thrombolytic treatment and prognosis of hemodynamically stable patients with major pulmonary embolism. Circulation 96:882–888
 4. Glassford DM, Akford WC Jr, Burrus GR et al (1981) Pulmonary embolectomy. Ann Thorac Surg 32:28–32
 5. Robison RJ, Fehrenbacher J, Brown JW et al (1986) Emergent pulmonary embolectomy: the treatment for massive pulmonary embolus. Ann Thorac Surg 42:52–55
 6. Kunieda T (1995) Acute fatal pulmonary thrombo-embolism. Kokyu to Junkan 43:873–879
 7. Meyer GT, Amisier D, Sors H et al (1991) Pulmonary embolectomy: a 20-year experience at one center. Ann Thorac Surg 51:232–236
 8. Mattox KL, Feldtman RW, Beall AC et al (1982) Pulmonary embolectomy for acute massive pulmonary embolism. Ann Surg 195:726–731
 9. Phillips SJ, Ballentine B, Slonine D et al (1983) Percutaneous initiation of cardiopulmonary bypass. Ann Thorac Surg 36:223–225
10. Vogel RA, Tommaso CL, Gundry SR (1988) Initial experience with coronary angioplasty and aortic valvuloplasty using elective semipercutaneous cardiopulmonary support. Am J Cardiol 62:811–813
11. Vogel RA (1988) The Maryland experience: angioplasty and valvuloplasty using percutaneous cardiopulmonary support. Am J Cardiol 162:11K–14K
12. Ohteki H, Suda H, Itoh T et al (1991) Percutaneous cardiopulmonary bypass: experimental and preliminary clinical use. Artifi Organs 14:62–64
13. Sakai M, Ohteki H, Doi K et al (1996) Clinical use of extracorporeal lung assist for patient in status asthmaticus. Ann Thorac Surg 62:885–887
14. Sakai M, Ohteki H, Doi K et al (1996) Clinical application and indications for percutaneous cardiopulmonary bypass support in cardiopulmonary failure of various etiologies. JJAAM 7:345–351

Surgical Treatment for Chronic Pulmonary Thromboembolism: Results from the Chiba University School of Medicine

MASAHISA MASUDA[1], KENJI MOGI[1], YOKO ONUKI[1], MITSURU NAKAYA[1], OSAMU OKADA[2], NOBUHIRO TANABE[2], TAKAYUKI KURIYAMA[2], and NOBUYUKI NAKAJIMA[1]

Summary. Chronic pulmonary thromboembolism is a frequent cause of progressive pulmonary hypertension and carries a poor prognosis. Medical treatment is not particularly effective, and surgery provides the only possibility of a cure at present. We report our experiences of surgical treatment for chronic pulmonary thromboembolism. Between June 1986 and February 1998, 35 patients underwent pulmonary surgical treatment at our hospital. Twelve patients (37.5%) had deep vein thrombosis. Our surgical indications were based on the San Diego group criteria. We have adopted two surgical approaches to pulmonary thromboendarterectomy. The preoperative mean pulmonary pressure was 46.7 ± 7.5 mmHg, the cardiac index was 2.41 ± 0.5 l/min per m^2, and the PVR was 901.3 ± 305.0 dyn·s·cm^{-5}. The PaO$_2$ (FiO$_2$ = 0.21) was 58.1 ± 8.5 mmHg. The number of operative deaths was six (17.1%). Twenty-nine patients survived, and the declines in their pulmonary arterial pressures and pulmonary vascular resistance, and the increases in their cardiac indices, were significant postoperatively. Their PaO$_2$ improved significantly after 6 months. We conclude that surgical treatment can improve the prognosis of patients with chronic pulmonary thromboembolism.

Keywords. Chronic pulmonary thromboembolism, Thromboendarterectomy, Median sternotomy approach, Lateral thoracotomy approach

Introduction

Chronic pulmonary embolism with pulmonary hypertension carries a particularly poor prognosis. Medical treatment is not effective, and surgical treatment provides the only potential cure at this time. We have operated on 35 cases of chronic pulmonary embolism since 1986. In this paper, we report our surgical experience and the follow-up results.

[1] First Department of Surgery and [2] Department of Chest Medicine, Chiba University School of Medicine, 1-8-1 Inohana, Chuo-ku, Chiba 260, Japan

Patients and Methods

Between June 1986 and February 1998, 35 patients (13 men, 22 women) underwent pulmonary thromboendarterectomy at our hospital. The mean age was 51.0 years (range 22–73). All patients complained of progressive dyspnea on effort of more than 6 months' duration (the mean interval from the onset of symptom to operation was 27.8 months). Thirty-three cases were in class III or IV of the classification of the New York Heart Association (NYHA) and III or IV of the Hugh-Johns classification. Twelve patients (37.5%) had deep vein thrombosis, and 10 patients (31.3%) had varicose veins of the lower extremities. The anticardiolipin antibody test was positive in six patients.

Our surgical indications were based on the San Diego group criteria as follows: (1) thrombi defined to be surgically accessible; (2) pulmonary vascular resistance (PVR) >300 dyne·s·cm^{-5}; (3) mean pulmonary arterial pressure (mPAP) >30 mmHg; (4) no life-threatening concomitant disease [1].

We have adopted two surgical approaches to pulmonary thromboendarterectomy. The first method is the unilateral thoracotomy approach (16 patients), and the other is the median sternotomy approach under cardiopulmonary bypass with deep hypothermia and intermittent circulatory arrest (14 patients), or with selective cerebral perfusion (5 patients). Our reasons for adopting the latter method were to obtain a good visibility without back bleeding from the bronchial artery, as well as to prolong the endarterectomy time while protecting against brain damage (Table 1).

Results

Preoperative Hemodynamics

The preoperative pulmonary hemodynamics data of all patients are shown in Table 2 and Fig. 1. The mean pulmonary pressure was 46.7 ± 7.5 mmHg, the

TABLE 1. Operative experience

	1986–1991	1992–1998
Number	14	21
Sex male	5	8
female	9	13
Mean age (years)	49 ± 14	52 ± 10
Mean PVR (dyne·s·cm^{-5})	860 ± 355	921 ± 271
Approach		
lateral thoracotomy	11	5
median with CPB	3	16
Mortality	3	3
Mortality rate	21.4%	14.3%

PVR, pulmonary vascular resistance; CPB, cardiopulmonary bypass.

cardiac index was 2.41 ± 0.5 l/min per m^2, and the PVR was 901.3 ± 305.0 dyne·s·cm^{-5}. The PaO$_2$ (FiO$_2$ = 0.21) was 58.1 ± 8.5 mmHg.

Surgical Results

As shown in Table 1, the number of operative deaths was six (17.1%). Three deaths were due to right ventricular failure with residual pulmonary hypertension because of inadequate thromboendarterectomy. Three additional patients died of postoperative severe pulmonary edema, pneumonia, and cardiac tamponade, respectively. One patient who was operated on under deep hypothermia with selective cerebral perfusion suffered a severe right cerebral embolism

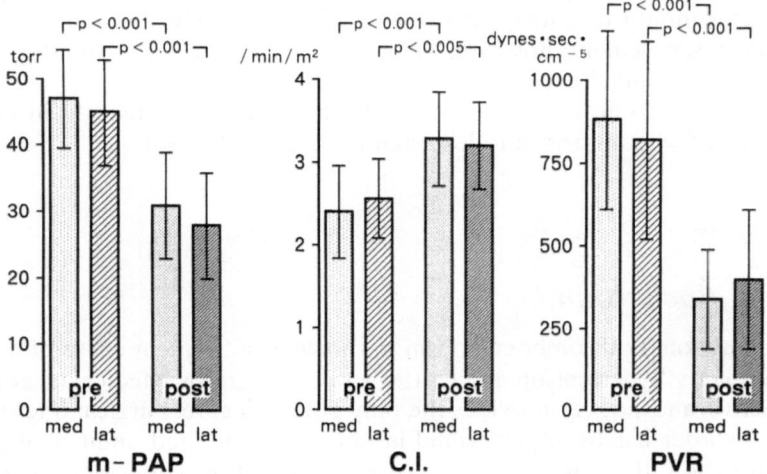

FIG. 1. Improvement of hemodynamics. The hemodynamic improvement was characterized by an immediate decrease of pulmonary arterial pressure and pulmonary vascular resistance (*PVR*) subsequent to an increase of cardiac output. Postoperative hemodynamic data between the median sternotomy approach and the lateral thoracotomy approach were not significant. *med*, median sternotomy approach; *lat*, lateral thoracotomy approach; *m-PAP*, mean pulmonary Arterial pressure; *C.I.*, cardiac index

TABLE 2. Hemodynamics and respiratory function

	Preop.	Postop.
mPAP (mmHg)	46.7 ± 7.5	28.7 ± 8.3
CI (l/min per m^2)	2.41 ± 0.50	3.25 ± 0.52
PVR (dyne·s·cm^{-5})	901.3 ± 305.0	375.6 ± 172.9
PaO$_2$ (room, mmHg)	58.1 ± 8.5	62.9 ± 11.3
PaCO$_2$ (room, mmHg)	34.5 ± 4.3	38.3 ± 3.43

mPAP, mean pulmonary arterial pressure; CI, cardiac index; PVR, pulmonary vascular resistance.

intraoperatively. However, the hemiplegia gradually improved, and she was able to be discharged. She can now take care of herself. Postoperative delirium was not observed in this series.

Of the median sternotomy approach patients, 4 of 19 (21.1%) died. Two of the 16 patients who underwent the thoracotomy approach (12.5 %) died.

Postoperative Hemodynamics

29 patients survived and were discharged from the hospital. The pulmonary hemodynamics data of the 29 patients are shown in Table 2. The declines in pulmonary arterial pressures and PVR and the rise in cardiac indices were significant. The hemodynamic change between the median approach group and the thoracotomy approach group was not significant. The blood gas analysis (FiO_2 = 0.21) after 1 month revealed a PaO_2 of 62.9 ± 11.3 mmHg, and did not show a significant improvement; however, PaO_2 increased to 76.9 ± 9.8 mmHg after 6 months, a significant change.

There was a significant improvement of symptoms after 6 months in 23 of 26 cases (88.5%) who improved to less than the NYHA II level.

Discussion

Surgical Background

Chronic pulmonary thromboembolism is known as a frequent cause of progressive pulmonary hypertension and carries a poor prognosis. Medical treatment is not effective, and surgery provides the only potential cure. Surgical intervention for this disorder has been performed in only a very limited number of institutions throughout the world [2, 3]. The largest series of thromboendarterectomies has been performed at the University of Calfornia, San Diego, which has done pioneering work in this procedure. In Japan, surgical management for this disease has been demonstrated to be effective in several reports since the first case was reported by Nakajima et al. in 1986 [4–6].

The natural history and poor prognosis of this disease were reported by Riedel and colleagues in 1982 [7]. In that report, they showed that patients with a mean pulmonary pressure over 30 mmHg had only a 30% chance of 5-year survival. The mean pulmonary pressure in our 35 cases was 46.7 mmHg, and all cases fell into the poor prognosis category.

Etiology

The etiology of chronic pulmonary thromboembolism remains unknown. Whether the failure to resolve emboli results from the deep vein thrombosis or from the pulmonary vascular endothelial change itself is uncertain. Abnormalities of protein C deficiency or anticardiolipin antibody deficiency were found in nine patients. We have experienced another two cases of pulmonary arterial stenosis caused by aortitis syndrome or solitary pulmonary arteritis [8].

In pulmonary thromboembolism (PTE), pulmonary hypertension progresses with time. This may be the result of recurrent embolic episodes or of a secondary thrombotic occlusion of the lumen.

Surgery

The specific preoperative evaluation includes right heart catheterization and pulmonary angiography [9]. Recently, we have attempted to diagnose and locate the lesions by angioscopy. Surgical indications were mentioned earlier. It is important to determine whether the lesion is accessible surgically. We are proposing that the localization of the lesion could be classified in three types according to pulmonary angiographic manifestations. These patterns are: (1) central, (2) central to peripheral, and (3) peripheral. They are illustrated in Fig. 2. According to this classification system, the thrombus formation originates in the main pulmonary artery and extends to the lobar artery in type 1. In type 2, the thrombus extends from the main pulmonary artery to the segmental or subsegmental arteries. In type 3, the occlusion of the lumen of the arteries is confined mainly to segmental or subsegmental arteries. From a surgical point of view, it is generally considered that types 1 and 2 are surgically or technically accessible, while type 3 is generally considered to be not technically feasible.

We have developed two surgical approaches for pulmonary thromboendarterectomy. The first is the median sternotomy approach, and the second is the thoracotomy approach. Most cases of PTE involve bilateral obstruction and pulmonary hypertension. Therefore, the median sternotomy approach is optimal. The layer for endarterectomy was so thin and fragile in some patients (Fig. 3) that we sometimes had to abandon this strategy. For this reason, we believe that the firmness may be different according to the duration from the onset to surgery (Fig. 4). We have adopted the median sternotomy approach as the standard

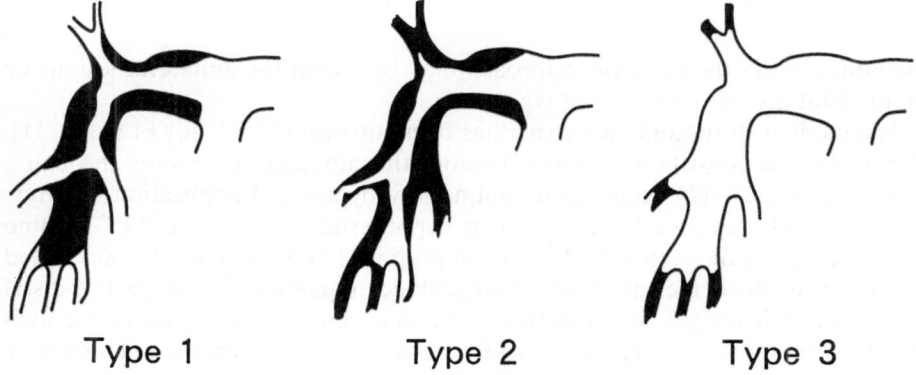

Type 1   Type 2   Type 3

FIG. 2. Morphological classification of steno-occlusive lesion of pulmonary arterial tree

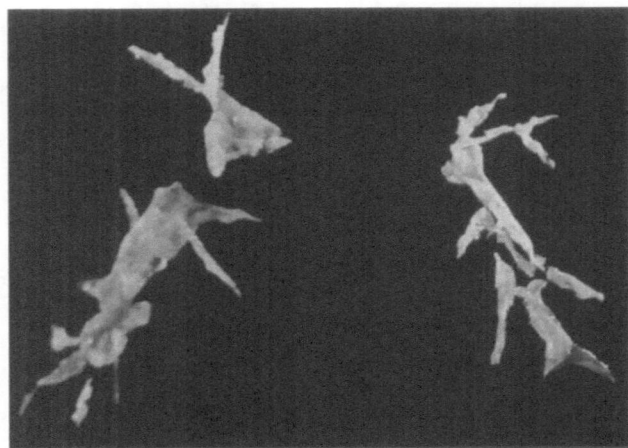

FIG. 3. The thromboen-
darterectomized
specimens from the
bilateral pulmonary
arteries were thin and
fragile

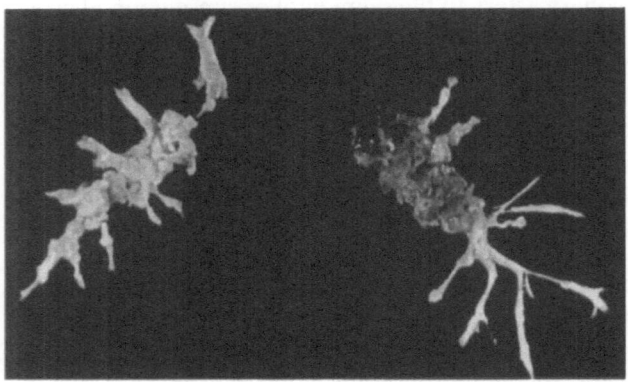

FIG. 4. This specimen was
very firm

method, but the thoracotomy approach may be useful for unilateral lesions or
more distal disease (peripheral type).

The median sternotomy approach has been advocated by Daily et al [10, 11].
This technique consists of: (1) simultaneous thromboendarterectomy through a
median approach, (2) under cardiopulmonary bypass, (3) application of intermittent circulatory arrest, and (4) deep hypothermia (at 18°C to 20°C). Some
modifications of the technique have been proposed by Jamieson, who succeeded
Daily in San Diego. He has reported surgical techniques for allowing better distal
visibility and leaving a rim of normal pulmonary artery at the level of the incision [12]. Moreover, as circulatory arrest times have been shortened in his series,
the incidence of postoperative delirium has decreased as well.

Fig. 5. Postoperative improvement of PaO$_2$. The PaO$_2$ did not immediately improve after operation, but significantly improved after 6 months

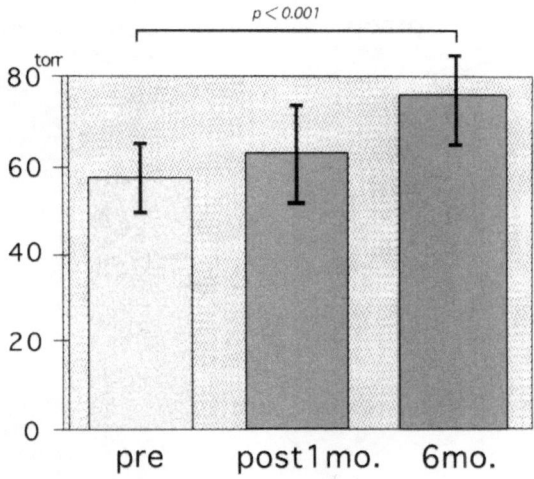

Surgical Results

The surgical results should be evaluated with regard to two different factors: surgical mortality, and hemodynamic and respiratory improvement.

The results obtained in our series demonstrated a marked improvement of hemodynamic and gas change, as reported in the literature [13]. The hemodynamic improvement was characterized by an immediate decrease of pulmonary artery pressure and PVR subsequent to an increase of cardiac output. The PaO$_2$ did not immediately improve after operation, but did improve during the follow-up period. The majority of patients did not require continuous oxygen therapy during the follow-up period. The marked hypoxemia in this disorder results from a perfusion-ventilation mismatch, decrease of cardiac output, and venous oxygen saturation. Postoperatively, reperfusion of the nonperfused area and an increase in cardiac output can be obtained, but it may take a certain amount of time for stabilization of the redistributed blood flow to occur. It is believed that pulmonary vascular steal and reperfusion pulmonary edema delay improvement in the PaO$_2$ level [14, 15] (Figs. 5,6).

Conclusion

We conclude that surgical treatment has improved the prognosis of patients with PTE. The beneficial effects on hemodynamics and gas exchange were confirmed. For further improvement of surgical outcomes, it is vitally important that medical and surgical teams interact for preoperative evaluation and postoperative management.

preop.   **postop. 1 month**   **6 months**

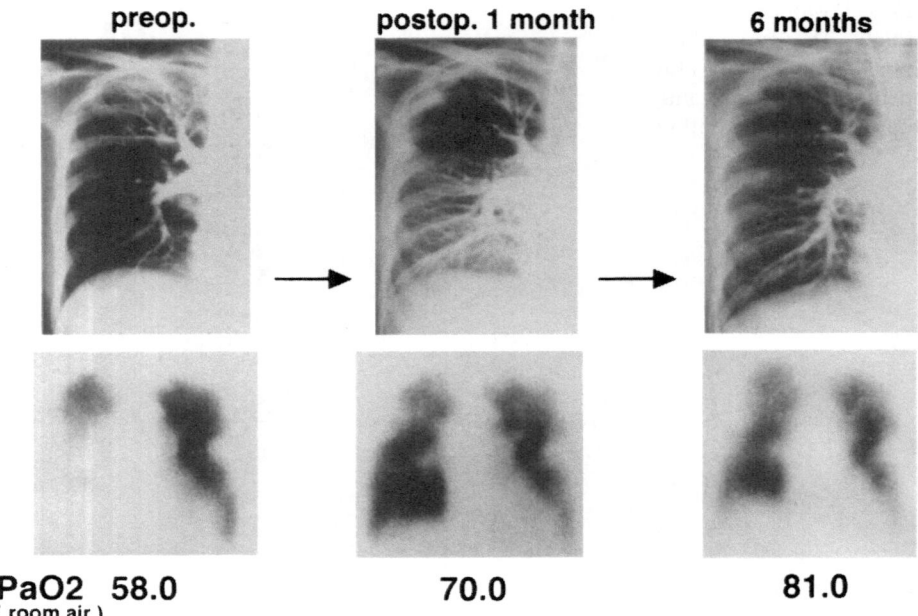

PaO2 58.0   **70.0**   **81.0**
(room air)

Fig. 6. Postoperative improvement of pulmonary angiographic findings and perfusion scans. These findings show it may take some time for stabilization of the redistributed blood flow

References

1. Jamieson SW, Auger WR, Fedullo PF et al (1993) Experiences and results with 150 pulmonary thromboendarterectomy operations over a 29-month period. J Thorac Cardiovasc Surg 108:116–127
2. Mayer E, Dahm M, Hake U et al (1996) Mid-term results of pulmonary thromboendarterectomy for chronic thromboembolic pulmonary hypertension. Ann Thorac Surg 61:1788–1792
3. Hartz RS, Byrne JG, Rich S et al (1996) Predictors of mortality in pulmonary thromboendarterectomy. Ann Thorac Surg 62:1255–1260
4. Nakagawa Y, Masuda M (1995) Surgical management for chronic pulmonary embolism: a review (in Japanese). Jpn J Phlebol 6:21–30
5. Nakajima N, Masuda M, Mogi K (1997) The surgical treatment for chronic pulmonary thromboembolism—our experience and current review of the literature. Ann Thorac Cardiovasc Surg 3:15–21
6. Nakajima N, Kawazoe K, Uemura S et al (1986) Experience of surgical treatment for chronic pulmonary thromboembolism (in Japanese). Jpn J Thorac Surg 34:524–531
7. Riedel M, Stanek V, Widimsky J et al (1982) Longterm follow-up of patients with pulmonary thromboembolism. Late prognosis and evolution of hemodynamic and respiratory data. Chest 81:151–158
8. Okubo S, Kunieda T, Nakajima N et al (1988) Idiopathic isolated pulmonary arteritis with chronic cor pulmonale. Chest 94:665–666

9. Auger WR, Fedullo PF, Moser KM et al (1992) Chronic major-vessel thromboembolic pulmonary artery obstruction: appearance at angiography. Radiology 182:393–398
10. Daily PO, Dembitsky WP, Iversen S (1989) Technique of pulmonary thromboendarterectomy for chronic pulmonary embolism. J Cardiac Surg 4:10–24
11. Daily PO, Dembitsky WP, Peterson KL et al (1987) Modifications of techniques and early results of pulmonary thromboendarterectomy for chronic pulmonary embolism. J Thorac Cardiovasc Surg 93:221–233
12. Jamieson SW (1995) Treatment of pulmonary hypertension due to chronic pulmonary thromboembolism. Phlebology 6:1–12
13. Fedullo PF, Moser KM (1997) Advances in acute pulmonary embolism and chronic pulmonary hypertension. Adv Intern Med 42:67–104
14. Olman MA, Auger WR, Fedullo PF et al (1990) Pulmonary vascular steal in chronic thromboembolic pulmonary hypertension. Chest 98:1430–1434
15. Tanabe N, Okada O, Nakagawa Y et al (1997) The efficacy of pulmonary thromboendarterectomy on long-term gas exchange. Eur Respir J 10:2066–2072

Current Status of Thromboendarterectomy for Chronic Pulmonary Embolism

PAT O. DAILY

Summary. Chronic pulmonary hypertension due to unresolved major vessel pulmonary emboli occurs infrequently but is extremely debilitating. The embolic material may be highly organized and thus resistant to fibrinolysis. A defect in the fibrinolytic system may also play a role in unresolved pulmonary emboli. Several embolic episodes may be necessary to cause chronic pulmonary vascular obstruction. The possibility of chronic pulmonary embolism should be considered in patients who present with chronic pulmonary hypertension. The definitive diagnosis depends on pulmonary arteriography. When pulmonary arteriography confirms the presence of proximally located major vascular obstruction, significant functional disability and pulmonary vascular resistance of at least 300 dynes·s·cm^{-5} are prerequisites for surgical consideration. Features of pulmonary thromboendarterectomy include median sternotomy, cardiopulmonary bypass with deep hypothermia and circulatory arrest, distal exposure of the orifices all the bronchopulmonary segmental arteries, and endarterectomy for areas of obstruction. Endarterectomy techniques are necessary because ingrowth of collagen and elastic tissue cause the organizing embolic material to adhere firmly to the pulmonary arterial wall within several weeks after acute embolization. The most recent data suggest that hospital mortality for pulmonary thromboendarterectomy is approximately 6% in the last 300 patients undergoing pulmonary thromboendarterectomy at the University of California, San Diego. In this group, over 90% of survivors were in New York Heart Functional Class I. In the next largest series published in the last 5 years, hospital mortality was 23% in 34 patients. Consequently, it is apparent that optimal results are based upon a highly experienced, multidisciplinary team dedicated to the management of these patients.

Keywords. Chronic pulmonary embolism, Pulmonary thromboendarterectomy

---

Sharp Memorial Hospital, 8010 Frost Street, Suite 501, San Diego, CA 92125, USA

Historical Perspective

As early as 1916 [1], it was suspected that chronic pulmonary embolism might lead to chronic pulmonary hypertension. However, the first proof of chronic pulmonary embolism was reported by Ljungdahl in 1928 [1]. There was over 50% obstruction of the pulmonary vasculature in two patients who died of progressive respiratory insufficiency. In 1950, the first confirmation of chronic pulmonary emboli causing severe pulmonary hypertension in living patients was reported by Caroll [2]. Hollister and Cull suggested endarterectomy as a method of removing chronically obstructive pulmonary emboli in 1956 [3]. However, technical problems prevented successful removal of the obstructive material. Hurwitt et al., in 1957 [4], attempted pulmonary endarterectomy with venal caval occlusion and hypothermia, but the patient died.

The first successful pulmonary endarterectomy was performed by Allison et al. in 1958 [5], using inflow occlusion and hypothermia. Snyder et al., in 1963 [6], reemphasized the adherent nature of the pulmonary embolus with respect to chronicity and were the first to employ endarterectomy techniques for removal of the obstructing material. Castleman et al. [7] reported that in 1964 Scannell et al. used cardiopulmonary bypass for pulmonary thromboendarterectomy and also reported hemorrhagic pneumonitis acutely following pulmonary thromboendarterectomy. In 1965, Moser et al. [8] reported four additional cases with two patients becoming long-term survivors.

In July 1970, Dr. Nina Braunwald performed the first pulmonary thromboendarterectomy at the University of California, San Diego which was reported in 1973 [9]. Subsequent series of pulmonary thromboendarterectomy at UCSD were reported by Daily et al. in 1980 [10], and Utley et al. in 1982 [11]. In a 1984 review, Chitwood et al. [1] reported 85 patients in the world literature who underwent pulmonary thromboendarterectomy. Thirty-three percent of these developed severe reperfusion pulmonary edema. The hospital mortality for the entire group was 22%. In 1987, Daily et al. [12] reported a series of modifications for improving the technique of pulmonary thromboendarterectomy in 41 patients. In the last group of that series, myocardial protection consisted of single-dose cardioplegia followed by application of a cooling jacket to keep the right and left ventricles at less than 10°C. There was no instance of phrenic nerve paresis and the operative mortality was 5.5%. The series was further extended to 127 patients by April of 1989 [13]. Risk factors for pulmonary insufficiency requiring long-term ventilation and death were the preoperative presence of ascites, the need for four units of blood or more, and the failure to obtain at least a 50% reduction of pulmonary vascular resistance intraoperatively. Subsequently, Jamieson et al. [14] reported an additional series of 150 pulmonary thromboendarterectomies at the University of California, San Diego, with an operative mortality of 8.7%. In 1997, the report by Fedullo and Moser [15] increased the number of patients undergoing pulmonary thromboendarterectomy at the University of California, San Diego to more than 700 with an overall operative mortality of 9.6%. In the last 300 patients, the operative mortality was 6.0%.

Incidence of Chronic Pulmonary Embolism

It is difficult if not impossible to arrive at the exact percentage of patients that develop chronic pulmonary hypertension following acute pulmonary embolism. In large part, this is due to the fact that there have been so many various estimates regarding the incidence of patients with acute pulmonary embolism that become chronic. For example, Bennotti et al. [16] surmised that perhaps 4.0% of patients were apt to become chronic with respect to persistent pulmonary hypertension. Paraskos et al. [17] suggested that cor pulmonale developed in only 2% of patients. A lesser number was proposed by Tilkian et al. [18], at 0.5%. In 1990, Moser [19] proposed an estimate of 0.1% which later in the same year was reestimated at 0.01% [20].

Since Dalen et al. [21] have suggested that 450000 patients per year survive acute pulmonary embolism, this leaves a range of 45 to 18000 patients per year that annually will potentially develop chronic pulmonary embolism. Considering the lower incidence of 0.01%, this would be only 45 patients per year in the United States that would develop chronic pulmonary embolism. As previously stated, Chitwood et al., in 1984 [1], were able to find only 85 patients in the world literature that had been surgically treated for chronic pulmonary embolism. Consequently, one would surmise that the diagnosis of chronic pulmonary embolism is considered infrequently. Furthermore, even currently, the therapeutic modality of pulmonary thromboendarterectomy for chronic pulmonary embolism is not considered sufficiently frequently. In some instances, heart–lung transplantation has been performed for chronic pulmonary embolism. Based upon the recent significant increase in the number of pulmonary thromboendarterectomies performed in a variety of centers in the United States, including over 700 patients at University of California, San Diego [15], it would seem that the incidence is somewhat higher than stated above. Probably a range of 0.1% to 1.0% is more accurate with respect to the incidence of chronic pulmonary embolism.

Pathogenesis

It is apparent that in a great majority of patients there is nearly complete resolution of vascular obstruction after acute massive pulmonary embolism [21]. For this reason, it has been suggested that a single episode of pulmonary embolism cannot lead to chronic obstruction. In fact, it is thought that multiple episodes of acute pulmonary embolism are necessary for chronic obstruction to occur [22]. The proof of this suggestion, though, has not been established. However, there are some factors that may be important in the pathogenesis of chronic pulmonary embolism. Certainly, one of these is the pathologic nature of the pulmonary emboli. For example, at the time of embolism some thrombi have become quite organized and are replaced to a great extent with fibrous tissue. Therefore, it would be difficult to imagine that lysis of these emboli could be significant. Furthermore, the fibrinolytic system may be compromised which would result in inadequate resolution of acute pulmonary embolism. In Fig. 1, an embolus is shown which is well formed, representing a virtual cast of the veins of origin. Also, there is a fibrous quality to these emboli. It is therefore likely that these emboli would not be well resolved by the fibrinolytic system. In Fig. 2, there is an embolus, removed for acute pulmonary embolism, that is relatively recent. This embolic material appears more susceptible to fibrinolysis.

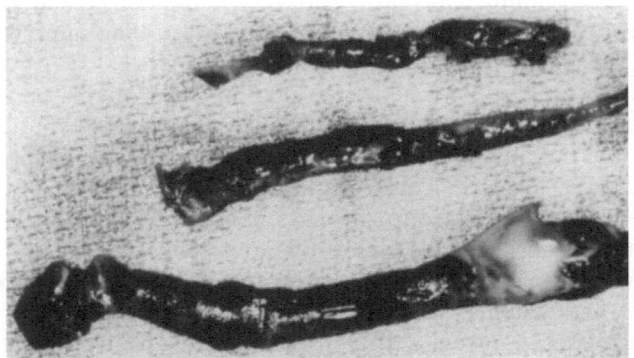

FIG. 1. These emboli appear to be well formed and have a fibrous quality. In the areas of discoloration, the emboli are particularly fibrous, suggesting they were older at the time of embolization and, therefore, the likelihood of fibrinolysis may be less. (From [44], with permission)

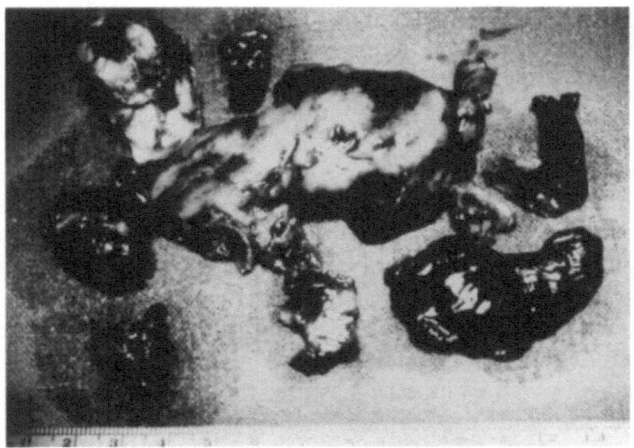

FIG. 2. Emboli removed from both pulmonary arteries. The emboli have the consistency and appearance of relatively recent thrombosis. Consequently, they would appear to be more susceptible to fibrinolysis. (From [44], with permission)

After acute pulmonary embolism, rapid changes occur within the pulmonary arteries that have been embolized. Figure 3 reveals the histological changes that occur 1 week after embolization. In fact, tissue ingrowth from the pulmonary artery into the embolus may occur as early as 3 days, attaching the pulmonary embolus to the pulmonary arterial wall. With additional time, the embolus becomes more firmly attached to the pulmonary arterial wall and subsequently can only be removed with pulmonary thromboendarterectomy techniques rather than simple pulmonary thromboembolectomy. As time progresses, the embolic material becomes replaced with both collagen and elastic tissue and is actually integrated into the wall of the pulmonary artery. The lumen then appears to resemble a normal pulmonary arterial lumen but is decreased in size. Because of these changes of attachment of the embolus to the pulmonary arterial wall, the embolic material cannot be removed by simple embolectomy. Therefore, endarterectomy methods must be employed [23]. This tendency of attachment of emboli to the pulmonary wall is further characterized in Fig. 4 which reveals that the intima and a portion of the media of the pulmonary arterial wall are removed at the time of thromboendarterectomy.

Indications for Pulmonary Thromboendarterectomy

The two most important factors for suggesting pulmonary thromboendar- terectomy are significant functional disability evidenced by New York Heart Functional Classification III or IV and the degree of pulmonary vascular resis- tance elevation. Based upon the data of Reidel and others [22], elevation of mean pulmonary artery pressure, of 30 mmHg or more, was associated with shortened

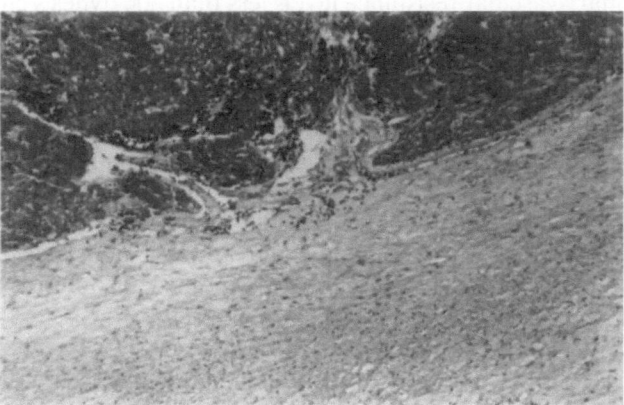

FIG. 3. Cross section of a pulmonary artery stained with hematoxylin and eosin at approx- imately 1 week after embolization. Significant ingrowth of fibrous tissue from the arterial wall into the embolus can be seen. Consequently, embolectomy by simple removal is no longer possible and thromboendarterectomy techniques are necessary

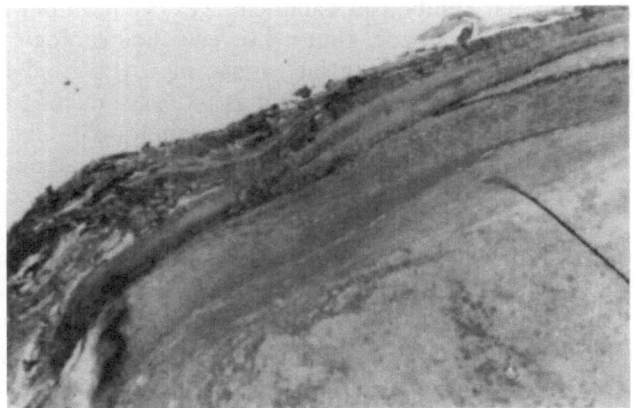

FIG. 4. This endarterectomy specimen reveals that the intima and a portion of the media have been removed with the organized embolus

survival. When the mean pulmonary artery pressure was greater than 50 mmHg, there was only a 10% 5-year survival. Although Reidel et al. [22] utilized mean pulmonary artery pressure, we found that a pulmonary vascular resistance of 300 dynes·s·cm^{-5} correlates quite well with 30 mmHg. An exception to the requirement of having at least 300 dynes·s·cm^{-5} or greater pulmonary vascular resistance is the relatively unusual occurrence of complete occlusion of either pulmonary artery. In these patients, pulmonary thromboendarterectomy results in considerable improvement of symptomatology even though the resistance may be less than 300 dynes·s·cm^{-5}. Additionally, there is a cohort of patients who may have pulmonary vascular resistance levels less than 300 dynes·s·cm^{-5} with rest, but with mild degrees of exertion have a rather marked elevation of pulmonary vascular resistance. These patients are also potential candidates for pulmonary thromboendarterectomy. Additionally, primary pulmonary hypertension must be distinguished from pulmonary artery occlusion or stenosis secondary to multiple embolization. Usually, the pulmonary arteriogram will allow distinction between chronic pulmonary embolism and primary pulmonary hypertension. Other entities that may be confused with chronic pulmonary embolism are primary pulmonary thrombosis without embolization and thrombosis secondary to underlying pulmonary hypertension [24]. Also, pulmonary thrombosis may occur with atrial septal defect [25].

Assuming that the degree of obstruction with respect to pulmonary vascular resistance has been met, the most important consideration in determining operability is the location of the beginning of the pulmonary arterial obstruction as determined by pulmonary angiography. Additionally, pulmonary artery endoscopy is increasingly utilized [15]. Ideally, the obstruction should begin in the main pulmonary arteries, but certainly proximal to the origins of the bronchopulmonary segmental arteries. If all of the obstructions are located distal to the apparent orifices of the bronchopulmonary segmental arteries, surgery should not be performed. The primary problem is that inadequate relief of pulmonary vascular resistance will occur, which markedly elevates the operative mortality [13].

Nicod et al. [26] and Auger et al. [27] have published details of pulmonary arteriography for chronic pulmonary embolism. The basic technique is to perform rapid-sequence large films in the AP view for the right side with the catheter positioned 5–7 cm into the right pulmonary artery. For the left side, the catheter is positioned similarly into the left main pulmonary artery, but in the left anterior oblique projection. Most commonly, these views are entirely adequate for establishing whether or not the patient is a potential operative candidate for pulmonary thromboendarterectomy. While pulmonary angioscopy [15, 28] has been suggested as an additional diagnostic tool, in some cases it is not possible to determine if endarterectomy can be performed. In fact, direct vision of the incised artery still does not allow precise determination of operability. In some instances, dissection has to be initiated before it is clear that a distinct plane of dissection can be obtained.

In summary, the pulmonary arteriogram is the preferred method of establishing the diagnosis of chronic pulmonary embolism as well as determining whether or not pulmonary thromboendarterectomy should be attempted. However, it is possible that in the future spiral computed tomography may allow less invasive methods for determination of operability [29].

Important Preoperative Considerations — Myocardial Protection

After the performance of bilateral pulmonary thromboendarterectomy, and even though most of the bronchopulmonary segments have been endarterectomized, there is often significant residual elevation of pulmonary vascular resistance. This resistance does decrease over additional time and usually to high–normal levels. Specifically, in a series of patients we reported [12], an intraoperative decrease of 59% in mean pulmonary vascular resistance occurred intraoperatively. Furthermore, Dittrich et al. [30] have described improved but not normal right ventricular function at follow-up. Consequently, myocardial protection is extremely important because of the persistent elevation in pulmonary vascular resistance after pulmonary thromboendarterectomy. For that reason, after a series of different methods, we now utilize maintenance of myocardial hypothermia with a cooling jacket which keeps all parts of the right and left ventricle and interventricular septum at 10°C or less [12, 13, 31]. Also, at the time of aortic cross-clamping, a single dose of cool blood cardioplegic solution of 1 liter is instilled through the ascending aorta. Utilizing this particular methodology for myocardial protection, the postoperative need for inotropic agents to maintain an adequate cardiac index has been minimized, and importantly, the right ventricle is well protected.

Circulatory Arrest

In the setting of chronic pulmonary thromboembolism, hypoxia gradually develops. The bronchial arteries hypertrophy in response to hypoxia. This is of significant technical importance at the time of pulmonary thromboendarterectomy in that once endarterectomy is started there is substantial bronchial back bleeding. In many cases, the back bleeding is so excessive that an adequate visual field cannot be maintained and intermittent circulatory arrest becomes necessary. Kirklin and Barrett-Boyes [32] have described that periods of circulatory arrest approaching 45 min are associated with significant permanent neurological defects. However, we have evolved the method of using periods of circulatory arrest for 20 min at a body temperature of 20°C or less. The period of 20 min of circulatory arrest is then followed by a 10-min period of reperfusion with arterial blood at less than 20°C [23].

Although postoperative delirium has been reported by Wragg et al.. [33], as characterized by agitation, hyperactivity, disorientation, and somnolence, we have seen no permanent neurologic defects. While the substantial majority of patients who undergo bilateral pulmonary thromboendarterectomy in well under a total of 60 min of circulatory arrest, we have on one occasion approached a total of 2 h of intermittent circulatory arrest with no neurological sequelae other than delirium. It is important to emphasize that delirium seems to have totally abated by the time of discharge from the hospital in essentially all patients. Recently, at the 1998 Society of Thoracic Surgeons meeting in New Orleans, Zund et al.. [34] reported a series of four patients who underwent bilateral pulmonary thromboendarterectomy with normal temperature (37°C) and continuous cardiopulmonary bypass. Presumably, no difficulties were encountered in performing the endarterectomies. Division of the superior vena cava facilitated exposure of the right pulmonary artery. Only four causes were reported, and there was no follow-up reported in this patient group.

Pulmonary Embolism Prophylaxis

It is essential in the postoperative period to prevent repeat pulmonary embolization. Therefore, if a vena caval filter has not been previously placed, it is usually accomplished 3 to 4 days prior to pulmonary thromboendarterectomy. At one point in time we were inserting the filter at the time of pulmonary thromboendarterectomy. However, to minimize the anesthetic time and to more precisely place a filter fluoroscopically, preoperative placement is preferred. Another essential aspect of prophylaxis for repeat embolism is the chronic administration of Coumadin for an indefinite period after the pulmonary thromboendarterectomy. Other anticoagulant modalities have not been attempted.

Surgical Technique

Prior to induction of anesthesia, a Swann-Ganz catheter is inserted through the right internal jugular vein. The tip of catheter is advanced 4–5 cm beyond the pulmonary valve so as to allow adequate determination of pulmonary artery pressure and at the same time not interfere with pulmonary thromboendarterectomy. The patient is positioned typically for median sternotomy with both lower extremities prepped and draped for the potential use of saphenous vein, if needed, for patch grafting of the pulmonary artery or coronary artery bypass grafting. If coronary artery bypass grafting is planned, the preferred donor vessels are the internal thoracic arteries since many patients have chronic venous disease. Cannulation of the ascending aorta is carried out followed by insertion of venous cannulae through the right atrium into the superior and inferior vena cava. Care is taken to ensure that superior vena caval cannula is placed well beyond the azygous vein. Cardiopulmonary bypass is then initiated and cooling is immediately started to 20°C. During the process of cooling, the superior vena cava is completely freed from its origin at the right atrium to the innominate vein. Posteriorly, the vena cava is freed in the area of the azygous vein. This allows manipulation of the superior vena cava to expose the right pulmonary artery. Next, the right pulmonary artery is dissected beginning at the pericardial reflection. Care is taken to dissect closely to the right pulmonary artery so as not to damage the right phrenic nerve. Typically, within a few minutes the heart fibrillates because of perfusion with blood at 20°C or less. At this point, umbilical tapes are placed around the superior and inferior vena cava to direct all venous return flow into the caval cannulae. A small incision is made in the right atrium which is carefully inspected for the presence of a patent foramen ovale and any thrombi or emboli. If any thrombi or emboli are identified, they are of course removed and the septal defect is either suture closed or patched, based on the size of the defect. As the patient's body temperature approaches 20°C, sodium thiamylal, phenytoin, and methylprednisolone are administered intravenously. It is also important to place a sump tube in the left atrium near the origin of the right superior pulmonary vein to minimize distention of the left ventricle. If the patient has significant aortic regurgitation, then as soon as ventricular fibrillation occurs from cooling, the aorta is cross-clamped and myocardial protection is carried out as previously described [12] except that the cardioplegic solution is delivered retrogradely through the coronary sinus.

In our experience, the electroencephalogram was continuously monitored, but in every instance when the above medications are administered and a blood temperature of 20°C or less is reached, the electroencephalogram is not recordable. Therefore, the electroencephalogram is no longer monitored routinely. Once the cardioplegic solution has been delivered, circulatory arrest is obtained. The venous drainage line is left open to remove as much blood as possible to minimize continued bleeding after endarterectomy is commenced. Initially, the incision is started in the right pulmonary artery inside the pericardial reflection and extended beyond the pericardial reflection to provide adequate access to the bronchopulmonary segmental branches of the middle and lower lobes (Fig. 8). The plane of dissection is started with a Penfield or neurosurgical elevator to define the correct plane (Fig. 9). Once the correct plane has been established, then dissection is performed with a variety of dissectors (see Figs. 5–7). The advantage of these dissectors is that suction can be applied continuously during dissection by virtue of a channel through the dissectors [35]. Even though circulatory arrest has been obtained, there is still significant back bleeding once dissection has started. Dissection is continued in a 360° circumferential

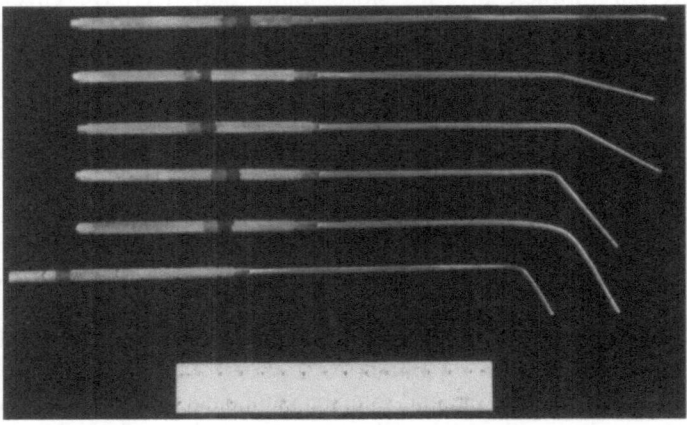

FIG. 5. Array of dissectors. The various angles of the dissectors and tip lengths facilitate dissection of all of the bronchopulmonary segmental arteries. The dimensions and angles are described in the text. (From [35], with permission)

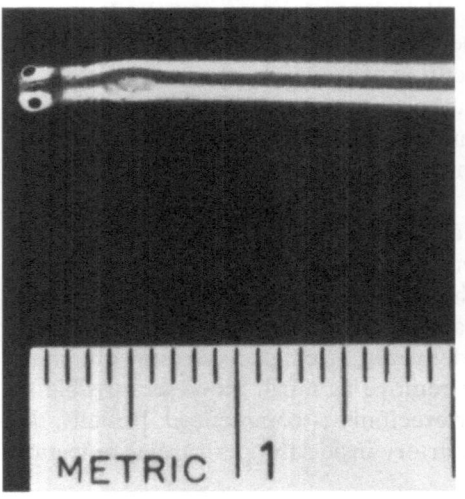

Fig. 6. Detail of dissector tips. The tip of the dissector is spherical and 2 mm in outside diameter. Four holes, 0.5 mm in diameter, are drilled at 90° to each other to permit simultaneous aspiration of blood during dissection. (From [35], with permission)

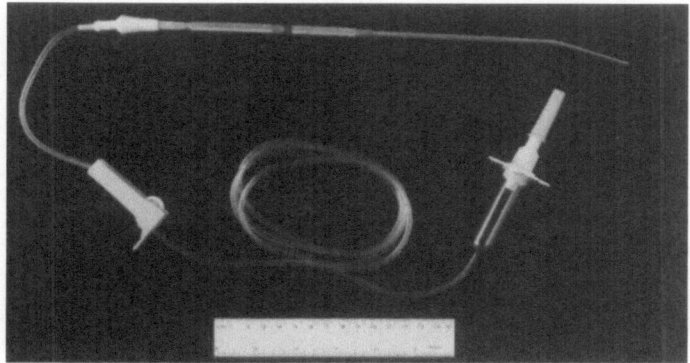

FIG. 7. Connection to intravenous (i.v.) tubing. A standard i.v. tubing is inserted into the end of the handle. The opposite end can be connected to wall suction, a cell saver device, or cardiotomy suction to conserve blood. (From [35], with permission)

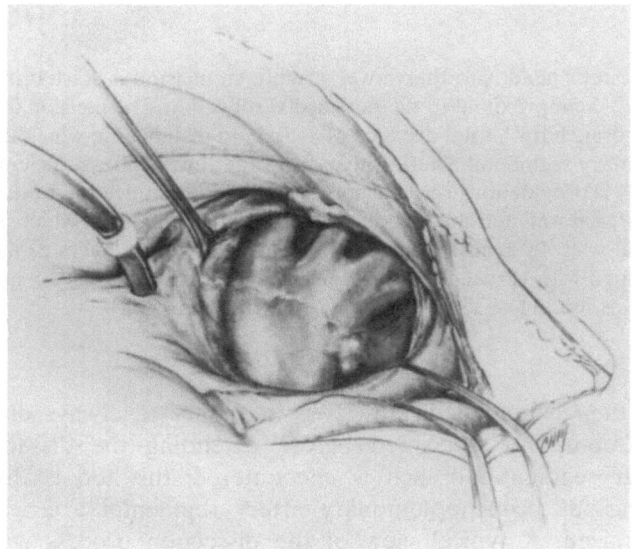

FIG. 8. The patient's head is to the viewer's right. The usual location of the extrapericardial right phrenic nerve is indicated. It is approximately 1 cm anterior to the right pulmonary artery. Therefore, incision of the pericardial reflection is made as close as possible to the right pulmonary artery. The incision is extended inferiorly to 1 cm below the right inferior pulmonary vein. Superiorly, the pericardial incision is extended 2 cm beyond the upper lobe branch. The line of reflection of the pericardium from the right pulmonary artery can be seen. Simultaneous with ventricular fibrillation, secondary to myocardial hypothermia, a left atrial sump tube is placed in the area of the right superior pulmonary vein. Inferior and lateral retraction of the right superior pulmonary vein enhances exposure of the right lower lobe pulmonary artery. The superior vena cava and aorta are retracted toward the patient's left by umbilical tapes. (From [23], with permission)

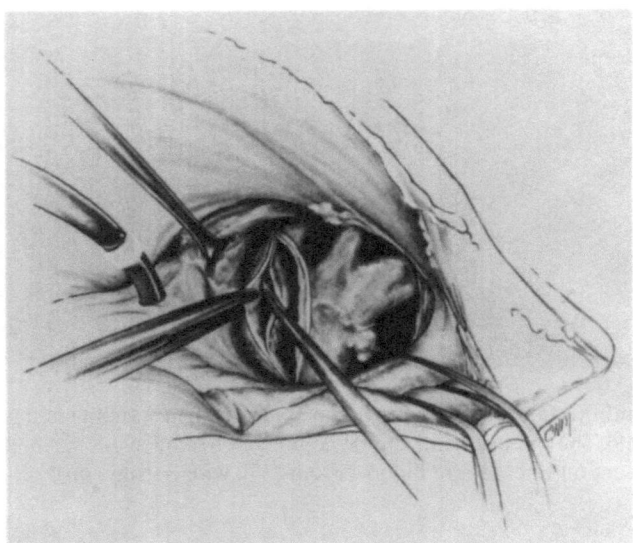

FIG. 9. The patient's head is to the viewer's right. An incision is started in the right pulmonary artery 2–3 cm proximal to the pericardial reflection. The incision is extended into the lower lobe branch for a total distance of 4–5 cm. In instances in which the middle lobe bronchopulmonary segmental arteries arise from the lower lobe, sufficient exposure for endarterectomy is provided. The critical consideration is identification of the correct plane between the arterial wall and the embolized but organized material which is incorporated into the arterial wall. To facilitate this identification, the outer layers of the arterial wall are gently grasped with vascular forceps, and dissection is started with a spatula and continued with an aspirating dissector. (From [23], with permission)

fashion and then extended distally. It is necessary to always dissect 360° to completely free-up the specimen before extending the dissection distally. Once another segmental branch is encountered, this too is dissected until all of the various bronchopulmonary artery segmental arteries have been endarterectomized. A typical view of the dissection process is seen in Fig. 10. As mentioned previously, after 20 min of circulatory arrest, cardiopulmonary bypass is reinstituted at 20°C or less for 10 min, and then again circulatory arrest is obtained and the cycle is repeated until each obstructed bronchopulmonary segmental artery has been endarterectomized. Once the right middle and lower lobes have been endarterectomized, it is possible at times to endarterectomize the upper lobe through the same incision. Alternatively, if adequate exposure is not obtained, a separate incision can be made in the superior aspect of the right pulmonary artery and continued into the right upper lobe branch, which facilitates endarterectomy of each bronchopulmonary segmental artery.

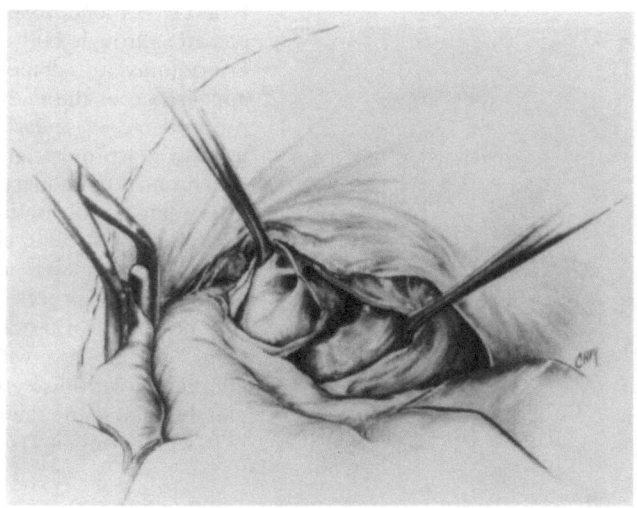

Fig. 10. The patient's head is to the viewer's left. As on the right side, the pericardial reflection is divided directly on the left pulmonary artery. This line of division extends inferiorly over the pulmonary veins to approximately 1 cm below the left inferior pulmonary vein. The incision is extended superiorly to 1 cm above the left pulmonary artery. A vein retractor is shown retracting the right superior pulmonary vein to the left and inferiorly. The left upper lobe bronchus can be visualized crossing anterior to the left pulmonary artery and posterior to the left superior pulmonary vein. The single incision in the pulmonary artery is started within the pericardial reflection and extended approximately 5 cm distally. It is important to extend the incision into the lower lobe branch and to avoid inadvertent extension of the incision into the upper lobe or lingular branches. If necessary, the incision can be extended 1.5–2.0 cm distal to the left upper lobe bronchus after the bronchus is dissected free from the pulmonary artery. If necessary, all eight bronchopulmonary segmental arteries of the left lung can be endarterectomized through the single incision as there were in the illustrated case. Typically, the left upper lobe and lingular branches are relatively spared and, therefore, they are not endarterectomized. (From [23], with permission)

During reperfusion the pulmonary arterial incisions may be closed with two rows of continuous 6–0 polypropylene suture.

For the left pulmonary artery a single incision is started intrapericardially and extended through the pericardium to the level of the upper lobe bronchus. The endoscopic appearance of the endarterectomy process is seen in Fig. 11.

As soon as the endarterectomy process is completed, rewarming to 37°C is initiated. If other surgical procedures are performed, such as coronary artery bypass grafting or valve replacement, they can be performed during cooling and/or rewarming. A typical surgical specimen is seen in Fig. 12. Frequently each bronchopulmonary segment is endarterectomized.

150   P.O. Daily

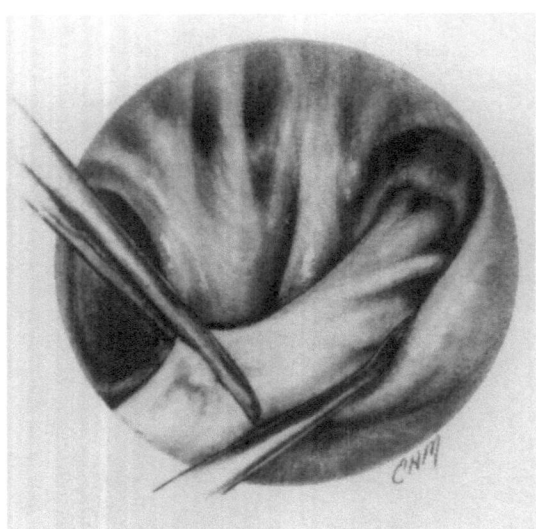

Fig. 11. An endoscope has been passed through the pulmonary arteriotomy to demonstrate the appearance of the endarterectomy process. A vascular forcep is used to grasp material obstructing the bronchopulmonary segmental artery and an aspirating dissector is passed distally 360° circumferentially. The specimen is grasped more distally and the process is repeated. It is necessary to use a hand-over-hand technique with forceps alternating with dissection to completely remove the material. (From [23], with permission)

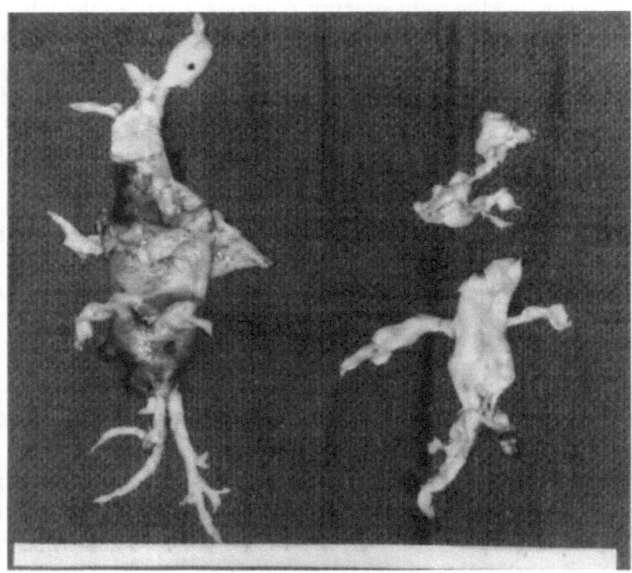

Fig. 12. Surgical specimen from pulmonary thromboendarterectomy of both pulmonary arteries. This specimen is oriented with the patient's right side to the viewer's left. Essentially all of the bronchopulmonary segmental arteries have been endarterectomized, resulting in a cast of the pulmonary arterial tree. (From [44], with permission)

Early Results

Chitwood et al.. [1] reported the first significant number of patients undergoing pulmonary thromboendarterectomy with respect to outcomes in 1984. They collected 85 patients reported in the world literature with an overall hospital mortality of 22%. In 1989, Jault and Cabrol [36] added 17 cases to the original 16 reported by Cabrol in 1978 [37]. In this group, the overall mortality was 20%. In the latter group of patients, pulmonary thromboendarterectomy was performed through a median sternotomy with bilateral thromboendarterectomy. However, deep hypothermia and circulatory arrest were not utilized. Although Moser and Braunwald [38] reported a single case of pulmonary thromboendarterectomy performed in 1970, the standardization of the surgical procedure began in February 1975. Extending to October 1983, 16 patients were operated on using cardiopulmonary bypass, deep hypothermia and circulatory arrest, and bilateral pulmonary thromboendarterectomy (see Table 2). The method of exposure in these patients was division of the pericardium so dissection could be carried outside the pericardial reflection, and this also allowed traction of the phrenic nerves for protection. Consequently, both pleural spaces were entered with this method. In this group of patients (group A), myocardial protection consisted of initiation of myocardial hypothermia with crystalloid cardioplegia and then maintenance of myocardial hypothermia with topical saline at 4°C, as described by Shumway et al.. [39].

A change in the methodology occurred in March 1984, and extended to September 1984, in a group of seven patients [12]. The methods of dissection and exposure of the pulmonary arteries were the same as in group A. However, the

TABLE 1. Survival related to mean pulmonary artery pressure

Mean pulmonary artery pressure (mmHg)	5-Year survival (%)
≦30	>90
31–40	45
41–50	35
≧50	10

Data from [22], with permission.

TABLE 2. Phrenic nerve paresis/mechanical ventilation support: hospital mortality and morbidity

Mean group	No. of patients	Hospital mortality rate[a]	Phrenic nerve paresis	Days on respirator
A (02/01/75–10/20/83)	16	3 (18.7%)	0 (0%)	8.4
B (03/12/84–09/11/84)	7	1 (14.3%)	5 (71%)	32.2
C (10/01/84–09/18/89)	149	17 (11.4%)	2 (1.34%)	4.5

Data from [12, 31], with permission.
[a] All deaths within 30 days or during hospitalization.

method of myocardial protection was the use of saline slush contained in a laparotomy pad. It was thought that containment of saline slush by the laparotomy pad would minimize the risk of phrenic nerve paresis. However, five of seven patients sustained phrenic nerve paresis of one or both phrenic nerves, necessitating prolonged ventilation of all patients. One death occurred in this group.

On October 1, 1984, the next significant changes resulted in modification of the methods of both myocardial protection and dissection. This group of patients is characterized as group C. In this group, after induction of myocardial hypothermia and cardiac arrest with cold blood cardioplegic solution, a cooling jacket was placed around the right and left ventricles for maintenance of myocardial hypothermia. Throughout the period of aortic cross-clamping, temperatures were measured at multiple sites. At all sites temperature was maintained at less than 10°C throughout the period of aortic cross-clamping [12]. The method of dissection was to initiate dissection of the pulmonary arteries inside the pericardium with distal extension of dissection beyond the pericardial reflection, but without entering the pleural spaces. The typical temperature curves for maintenance of myocardial hypothermia in multiple sites are seen in Fig. 13.

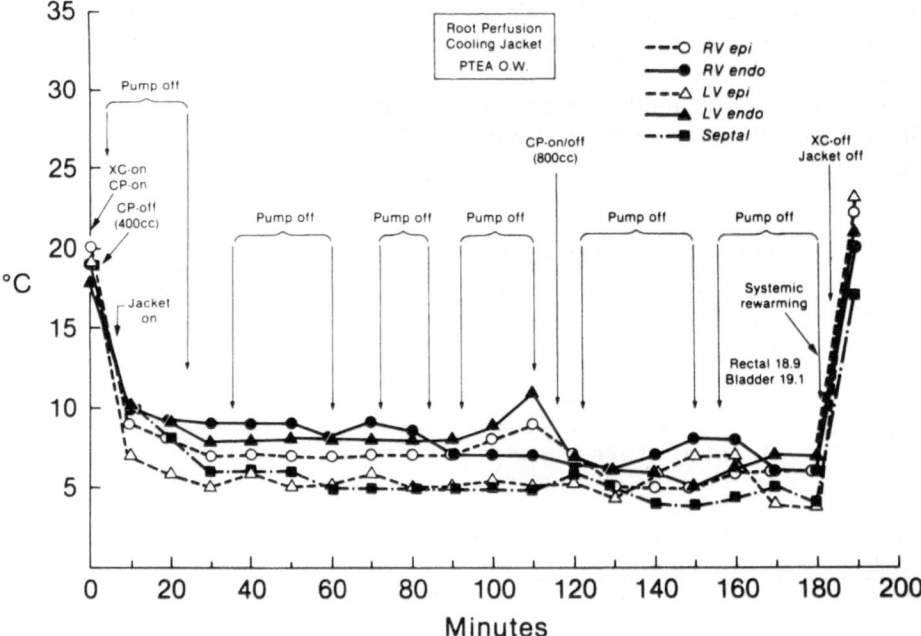

FIG. 13. Myocardial temperature curves during cardiac ischemia. This patient had the longest cross-clamp time in the entire series (186 min). All myocardial temperatures are consistently maintained at 10°C or less. *PTEA* pulmonary thromboendarterectomy; *RV*, right ventricular; *LV*, left ventricular; *Epi*, epicardium; *Endo*, endocardium; *XC*, cross-clamp; *CP*, cardioplegia. (From [44], with permission)

This latter group of 149 patients, extending to September 1989 [31], was analyzed in more detail. Reperfusion pulmonary edema necessitating the need for prolonged ventilation was by far the most significant complication (see Table 3). Ventilatory dependency was defined as the need for mechanical ventilation for a period of 5 days or more. Other complications are characterized in Table 4. A number of factors were analyzed using multivariate analysis of the causes of ventilator dependency and hospital mortality. These factors are summarized in Table 5. Independent predictors of ventilator dependency were the presence of preoperative ascites, total cardiopulmonary bypass time, and the need to administer more than 4 units of blood. Failure to lower the pulmonary vascular resistance by more than 50% nearly reached statistical significance. Hospital mortality was predicted by prolonged cardiopulmonary bypass time and the failure to lower the pulmonary vascular resistance by more than 50%. Moser et al.. reported an update of the late results of pulmonary thromboendarterectomy in 1990 [40]. These results are summarized in Tables 6 and 7. The most significant change was the decrease in pulmonary vascular resistance from 997 ± 624 dynes·s·cm^{-5}

TABLE 3. Causes of death

Cause of Death	Total no. of deaths		Postoperative day(s)
	No.	Percent	
Respiratory and multi-organ failure	10	58.8	19.9; range, 4–47
Pulmonary hemorrhage	3	17.6	1; range, 0–3
Acute myocardial infarction	1	5.9	3
Right heart failure[a]	1	5.9	0
Pulmonary artery thrombosis	1	5.9	6
Late cardiac tamponade	1	5.9	17

Data from [31], with permission.
[a] Intraoperative deaths.

TABLE 4. Complications

	No. of patients[a]	Percent
New myocardial infarction	2	1.6
Reintubation	1	0.8
Tracheostomy	6	4.8
Phrenic nerve paresis (transient)	1	0.8
Pneumonia (+ culture)	19	15.3
Sternal wound infection	6	4.8
Sepsis (+ blood culture)	9	7.2
Bleeding requiring reoperation	7	5.6
Postoperative low cardiac output cardiac index <2.0, >6 h)	6	4.8
Focal cerebral deficit	5	4.0
Requiring dialysis	5	4.0
No. of days in hospital (hospital survivors)	19.8 ± 12.5	(2–71)

Data from [13], with permission.
[a] $n = 124$; intraoperative deaths excluded.

TABLE 5. Multivariate analysis ($n = 124$)[a]

Variables	Ventilator dependency				Mortality			
	All patients $n = 39$		Hospital survivors $n = 28$		Total mortality $n = 16$		Respiratory failure $n = 12$	
	Coef.	P-value	Coef.	P-value	Coef.	P-value	Coef.	P-value
Ascites	1.2444	0.0008	1.4539	0.0002	–	–	–	–
Total bypass time	0.0114	0.0342	0.0119	0.0350	0.0121	0.0015	–	–
More than 4 blood product units	0.4898	0.0397	–	–	–	–	–	–
Percent change in pulmonary vascular resistance ≤50%	0.4671	0.0880	–	–	1.1980	0.0001	1.5688	0.0001
Preoperative pulmonary vascular resistance	–	–	–0.0256	0.0546	–	0.0016	–	0.0912
Constant	–1.6050	–	–0.2959	–	–4.5231	–	–3.3661	–

From [13], with permission.
[a] Intraoperative deaths excluded.

TABLE 6. Hemodynamics ($n = 34$)

Parameter	Preoperative	Immediate postoperative	Follow-up[a]
Mean pulmonary artery pressure (mmHg)	48.5 ± 12.4	26.6 ± 7.5*	24.3 ± 10.0
Cardiac output (l/min)	3.82 ± 1.29	5.92 ± 1.15*	4.85 ± 1.01*
Pulmonary vascular Resistance (dynes·s·cm^{-5})	997 ± 624	230 ± 110*	272 ± 256

Data from [20], with permission.
[a] Time of follow-up: 3 months to 16 years.
* $P < 0.05$ compared with immediate postoperative value; values are given as mean ± SD.

to 272 ± 256 dynes·s·cm^{-5} at follow-up extending from 3 months to 16 years. The level of pulmonary vascular resistance is comparable to long-term survival reported by Reidel et al.. [22]. Hartz et al.. [41] also evaluated predictors of mortality in a group of 34 patients undergoing pulmonary thromboendarterectomy. Overall, the operative mortality was 23%. However with preoperative pulmonary vascular resistance greater than 1100 dynes·s·cm^{-5}, and a mean pulmonary artery pressure more than 50 mmHg, the operative mortality was seven times higher than those patients with a lesser level of pulmonary vascular obstruction (41% vs 6%).

Current early results reported by Daily et al.. [31] suggest that long-term survival is improved. Specifically, at 1 year after pulmonary thromboendarterectomy the survival rate was 85% compared with 50% for heart–lung or lung transplantation. With an operative mortality of 25% or more for heart–lung transplanta-

TABLE 7. New York Heart Association
functional classification ($n = 117$)

Class	Preoperative	Postoperative[a]
I	0	85
II	5	26
III	49	6
IV	63	60

Data from [45], with permission.
[a]Follow-up $\geqq 1$ year.

tion, it is only logical to suggest pulmonary thromboendarterectomy rather than pulmonary transplantation as a primary treatment mode for chronic obstruction of the pulmonary arteries secondary to embolization [42]. However, in obtaining these results it is essential to carefully select patients with more proximally located thromboembolic obstructions. If these obstructions appear to be more distally located as assessed by pulmonary arteriography, then lung or heart–lung transplantation may be indicated as a primary procedure. However, as suggested by Shure [43], unanswered questions regarding pulmonary thromboendarterectomy persist.

References

1. Chitwood WR, Sabiston DC, Welchsler AS (1984) Surgical treatment of chronic unresolved pulmonary embolism. Clin Chest Med 5:507–536
2. Carroll D (1950) Chronic obstruction of major pulmonary arteries. Am J Med 9:175–185
3. Hollister LE, Cull VL (1956) The syndrome of chronic thrombosis of the major pulmonary arteries. Am J Med 21:312–320
4. Hurwitt ES, Schein CJ, Rifkin H et al (1958) A surgical approach to the problem of chronic pulmonary artery obstruction due to thrombosis or stenosis. Ann Surg 147:157–165
5. Allison PR, Dunnill MS, Marshall R (1960) Pulmonary embolism. Thorax 15:273–83
6. Snyder WA, Kent DC, Baisch BF (1963) Successful endarterectomy of chronically occluded pulmonary artery: clinical report and physiologic studies. J Thorac Cardiovasc Surg 45:482–489
7. Castleman B, McNeeley, Scannell G (1964) Case records of the Massachusetts General Hospital, Case 32-1964. N Engl J Med 271:40–50
8. Moser KM, Houk VN, Jones RC et al (1965) Chronic, massive thrombotic obstruction of pulmonary arteries: analysis of four operated cases. Circulation 32:377–385
9. Moser KM, Braunwald NS (1973) Successful surgical intervention in severe chronic thromboembolic pulmonary hypertension. Chest 64:29–35
10. Daily PO, Johnston GG, Simmons CJ et al (1980) Surgical management of chronic pulmonary embolism. J Thorac Cardiovasc Surg 79:523–531
11. Utley JR, Spragg RG, Long WB et al (1982) Pulmonary endarterectomy for chronic obstruction: recent surgical experience. Surgery 92:1096–1102

12. Daily PO, Dembitsky WP, Peterson KL et al (1987) Modification of techniques and early results of pulmonary thromboendarterectomy for chronic pulmonary embolism. J Thorac Cardiovasc Surg 93:221–233
13. Daily PO, Dembitsky WP, Iversen S (1990) Risk factors for pulmonary thromboendarterectomy. J Thorac Cardiovasc Surg 99:670–678
14. Jamieson SW, Auger WR, Fedullo PF et al (1983) Experience and results with 150 pulmonary thromboendarterectomy operations over a 29-month period. J Thorac Cardiovasc Surg 106:116–127
15. Fedullo PF, Moser KM (1997) Advances in acute pulmonary embolism and chronic pulmonary hypertension. Adv Intern Med 42:67–104
16. Bennotti JR, Ockene IS, Alpert JS et al (1983) The clinical profile of unresolved pulmonary embolism. Chest 84:669–678
17. Paraskos JA, Adelstein SJ, Smith RE et al (1973) Late prognosis of acute pulmonary embolism. N Engl J Med 298:55–58
18. Tilkian AG, Schroeder JS, Robin ED (1967) Chronic thromboembolic occlusion of main pulmonary artery or primary branches. Am J Med 60:563–573
19. Moser KM (1990) Venous thromboembolism. Am Rev Respir Dis 141:235–249
20. Moser KM, Auger WR, Fedullo PF (1990) Chronic major-vessel thromboembolic pulmonary hypertension. Circulation 81:1735–1743
21. Dalen JE, Banas JS, Brooks HL et al (1969) Resolution rate of acute pulmonary embolism in man. N Engl J Med 280:1194–1199
22. Reidel M, Stanek V, Widimsky J et al (1982) Long term follow-up of patients with pulmonary thromboembolism. Late prognosis and evolution of hemodynamic and respirator data. Chest 81:151–158
23. Daily PO, Dembitsky WP, Iversen S (1989) Technique of pulmonary thromboendarterectomy for chronic pulmonary embolism. J Card Surg 4:10–24
24. Yamaki S, Horiuchi T, Miura M et al (1989) Pulmonary vascular disease in secundum atrial septal defect with pulmonary hypertension. Chest 89:694–698
25. Schamroth CL, Sareli P, Pocock WA et al (1987) Pulmonary arterial thrombosis in secundum atrial septal defect. Am J Cardiol 60:1152–1156
26. Nicod P, Peterson KM, Levine MS et al (1987) Pulmonary angiography in severe chronic pulmonary hypertension. Ann Intern Med 107:565–568
27. Auger WR, Fedullo, Moser KM et al (1992) Chronic major vessel thromboembolic pulmonary artery obstruction: appearance at angiography. Radiology 182:393–398
28. Shure D, Gregoratos G, Moser KM (1985) Fiberoptic angioscopy: role in the diagnosis of chronic pulmonary arterial obstruction. Ann Intern Med 103:844–850
29. Roberts HC, Kauczor HU, Schweden F et al (1997) Spiral CT of pulmonary hypertension and chronic thromboembolism. J Thorac Imag 12(2):118–127
30. Dittrich HC, Chow LC, Nicod PH (1989) Early improvement in left ventricular diastolic function after relief of chronic right ventricular pressure overload. Circulation 80:823–830
31. Daily PO, Dembitsky PO, Iversen S et al (1990) Current early results of pulmonary thromboendarterectomy for chronic pulmonary embolism. Eur J Cardiothorac Surg 4:117–123
32. Kirklin JW, Barrett-Boyes BG (1986) Cardiac surgery. Morphology, diagnostic criteria, natural history, techniques, results, and indications. Wiley, New York, pp 42–43
33. Wragg RE, Dimsdale JE, Moser KM et al (1988) Operative predictors of delirium after pulmonary thromboendarterectomy. A model for postcardiotomy delirium? J Thorac Cardiovasc Surg 96:524–529

34. Zund G, Pretre R, Iselin D et al (1998) New approach for surgical management of chronic pulmonary embolism. Presented at the 1998 Society of Thoracic Surgeons meeting in New Orleans, LA, USA, by invitation
35. Daily PO, Dembitsky WP, Daily RP (1991) Dissectors for pulmonary thromboendarterectomy. Ann Thorac Surg 51:842–843
36. Jault F, Cabrol C (1989) Surgical treatment for chronic pulmonary thromboembolism. Herz 14:192–196
37. Cabrol C, Cabrol A, Acar J et al (1978) Surgical correction of chronic postembolic obstructions of the pulmonary arteries. J Thorac Cardiovasc Surg 76:620–628
38. Moser KM, Braunwald NS (1973) Successful surgical intervention in severe chronic thromboembolic pulmonary hypertension. Chest 64:29–35
39. Shumway NE, Lower RR, Stofer RC (1959) Selective hypothermia of the heart in anoxic cardiac arrest. Surg Gynecol Obstet 109:750–754
40. Moser KM, Auger WR, Fedullo PF (1990) Chronic major-vessel thromboembolic pulmonary hypertension. Circulation 81:1735–1743
41. Hartz RS, Byrne JG, Levitsky S et al (1996) Predictors of mortality in pulmonary thromboendarterectomy. Ann Thorac Surg 62:1255–1260
42. Dembitsky WP, Daily PO, Moser KM et al (1989) Pulmonary thromboendarterectomy as the preferred alternative to heart-lung transplantation for chronic pulmonary embolism. In: Belfus (ed) Cardiac surgery: state of the art reviews. Hanley and Belfus, pp 577–582
43. Shure D (1996) Thromboendarterectomy: some unanswered questions. Ann Thorac Surg 62:1253–1254
44. Daily PO (1990) Surgical management of chronic pulmonary embolism. In: Bergan JJ, Yao JST (eds) Venous disorders. Saunders, Philadelphia, pp 542–554
45. Fedullo PF, Auger WR, Channick RN et al (1995) A multidisciplinary approach to chronic thromboembolic pulmonary hypertension. In: Atlas of heart diseases 3:7.1–7.25

Prevention

Low Molecular Weight Heparins

C. Gregory Elliott

Summary. A large and growing body of scientific evidence exists which suggests that low molecular weight heparins are at least as effective and safe as other anti-coagulants used to treat and prevent venous thromboembolism. Low molecular weight heparins offer important advantages over unfractionated heparin for the treatment of venous thromboembolism. Low molecular weight heparins can be dosed according to the patient's weight, and monitoring of anticoagulant response is not necessary. For this reason, selected patients with deep vein thrombosis can be managed without hospitalization. The use of low molecular weight heparins to prevent venous thrombosis and pulmonary embolism depends upon costs, relative risks and benefits for specific indications, and additional scientific studies which address unanswered or incompletely answered questions, such as whether preoperative dosing is superior to postoperative dosing.

Keywords. Low molecular weight heparin, Deep vein thrombosis, Pulmonary embolism

Introduction

More than 25 years of basic and clinical investigation have shown that low molecular weight heparins are effective and safe for the prevention and treatment of venous thromboembolism. Low molecular weight heparins provide physicians with an alternative to unfractionated heparin and coumadin. The degree to which physicians use low molecular weight heparins will depend upon a complex balance of outcomes and costs. This chapter provides an overview of available data.

Pulmonary Divisions and Departments of Medicine, LDS Hospital and University of Utah School of Medicine, Salt Lake City, UT 84143, USA

Comparison of Biochemistry and Pharmacology of Low Molecular Weight Heparins and Unfractionated Heparin

Unfractionated heparin is a glycosaminoglycan which consists of chains of D-glucosamine and uronic acid residues. It ranges in molecular weight from 3000 to 30000. In contrast, low molecular weight heparins are fragments of unfractionated heparin produced by enzymatic or chemical depolymerization. The mean molecular weights of these fragments range from 4200 to 6000 (Table 1), and individual low molecular weight heparins are unique with respect to biologic behavior [1].

Unfractionated heparin differs fundamentally from low molecular weight heparins with respect to protein and cell binding [2, 3]. Heparin binds to endothelial cells and macrophages [4], whereas low molecular weight heparins do not. Heparin clearance is dose dependent and has two phases: (1) a rapid saturable phase and (2) a slow first-order mechanism [5]. Low molecular weight heparin clearance is dose dependent because molecules do not bind to cells and proteins. Low molecular weight heparin clearance is 2- to 4-fold slower than unfractionated heparin. Low molecular weight heparins are excreted by the kidneys, and low molecular weight heparin half-life increases in patients with renal failure [6].

In animal models, prevention of experimental venous thrombosis with low molecular weight heparin occurs at anti-Xa levels of 0.2 to 0.3 units/ml. Concentrations of 0.7 anti-Xa units/ml are necessary to inhibit growth of established thrombus. Bleeding from standardized animal injuries is more severe with unfractionated heparin than low molecular weight heparin at equivalent antithrombotic doses [7]. This may reflect effects of heparin on platelets [8].

Treatment of Symptomatic Deep Vein Thrombosis

Inpatient Therapy

Well-designed clinical trials have established the effectiveness and safety of low molecular weight heparins for the treatment of acute deep vein thrombosis (Table 2). A number of trials have shown that low molecular weight heparins

TABLE 1. Low molecular weight heparin preparations

Generic name	Trade name	Mean molecular weight	Anti-Xa/ IIa ratio
Ardeparin	Normiflo	6000	1.9
Dalteparin	Fragmin	6000	2.7
Enoxaparin	Lovenox	4200	3.8
Nadroparin	Fraxiparine	4500	3.6
Reviparine	Clivarin	4000	3.5
Tinzaparin	Innohep	4500	1.9

TABLE 2. Clinical trials which compare low molecular weight heparins (LMWH) with unfractionated heparin (UH) for treatment of acute deep vein thrombosis

First author, year [Ref.]	LMWH	Dose anti-Xa units[a]	Recurrence rate (%)		Major bleeding rate (%)		Mortality (%)	
			LMWH	UH	LMWH	UH	LMWH	UH
Hull, 1992 [12]	Tinzaparin	175/kg qd	2.8	6.9	0.5*	5.0	4.7	9.6
Columbus, 1997 [17][b]	Reviparin	6300 b.i.d. (>60 kg) or 4200 b.i.d. or 3500 b.i.d.	5.3	4.9	3.1	2.3	7.1	7.6
Levine, 1996 [15]	Enoxaparin	1 mg/kg b.i.d.	5.3	6.7	2.0	1.2	4.4	6.7
Koopman, 1996 [16]	Nadroparin	4100 or b.i.d. 6150 based on weight	6.9	8.6	0.5	2.0	6.9	8.1
Fiessinger, 1996 [29]	Dalteparin	200/kg qd	4.2	2.3	0.0	1.5		

[a] Includes patients with symptomatic pulmonary embolism and patients with prior deep vein thrombosis.
[b] All doses were administered subcutaneously.
* Significantly different ($P < 0.01$).

prevent thrombus growth more effectively than unfractionated heparin [9–11]. In these trials, venograms and lung scans were repeated after initial treatment to detect asymptomatic thrombus or thromboembolism.

Subsequent clinical trials examined clinical endpoints, including symptomatic recurrent venous thromboembolism [12]. A randomized double-blind clinical trial which compared continuous intravenous unfractionated heparin with once daily subcutaneous low molecular weight heparin (tinzaparin) showed fewer symptomatic recurrent venous thrombi and pulmonary emboli, and a significant reduction in major bleeding complications accompanied the use of tinzaparin [12]. In this trial, symptomatic recurrent thromboemboli occurred in 7% of 219 patients who received unfractionated heparin; whereas only 3% of 213 patients treated with low molecular weight heparin had recurrent venous thromboemboli during 3 months' follow-up ($P = 0.07$). In addition, 5% of those patients who were treated with unfractionated heparin developed major bleeding complications, whereas only 0.5% of 213 patients treated with low molecular weight heparin had major bleeding complications ($P = 0.006$).

Furthermore, treatment with tinzaparin was more cost effective than treatment with unfractionated heparin [13]. Estimates, based upon actual costs at the time of this clinical trial, suggested a savings of US$40149 for the treatment of 100 inpatients [13]. Savings were realized because of reduced costs for managing recurrent thromboembolism and major bleeding complications, as well as reduced costs for monitoring the anticoagulant effect of unfractionated heparin. Cost savings may be offset if the charges for low molecular weight heparins are high. However, additional cost savings are likely when low molecular weight heparins are used to treat patients without hospitalization.

Because individual low molecular weight heparins differ, other clinical trials have compared dalteparin [14], enoxaparin [9, 15], nadroparin [16], and reviparin [17] with unfractionated heparin for the treatment of symptomatic acute deep vein thrombosis. Although differences exist in the design of these clinical trials, each trial has shown that low molecular weight heparin is at least as effective and safe as unfractionated heparin. When investigators combine data from these trials and perform formal meta-analyses, they report significant reductions in the rates of recurrent thromboembolism, major bleeding, and mortality [18].

Predictable dosing is a major advantage of low molecular weight heparins. The physician-investigators used either weight-adjusted dosing (e.g., 175 anti-Xa units/kg [12]) or fixed doses (e.g., 6300 anti-Xa units twice daily) for patients weighing more than 60 kg [17]. These doses were given either once or twice each day by subcutaneous injection. Laboratory monitoring (e.g., activated partial thromboplastin time (aPTT) tests) and dose adjustments were not needed. The advantage of predictable dosing without laboratory monitoring, coupled with the proven efficacy and safety of low molecular weight heparins for inpatient therapy of deep vein thrombosis, made outpatient treatment of deep vein thrombosis feasible.

Outpatient Therapy

Two major clinical trials have suggested that low molecular weight heparins are effective and safe for outpatient treatment of selected patients with acute deep vein thrombosis [15, 16]. In one trial, Koopman et al. [16] compared nadroparin with unfractionated heparin. In this trial, patients randomly assigned to receive nadroparin who were willing and able to be treated at home either were not admitted to the hospital (36%) or were discharged early (40%). Importantly, this trial excluded patients with suspected pulmonary embolism. Only 81% of patients treated with heparin had attained a therapeutic aPTT within the first 24 h of treatment. With this caveat, the rates of recurrent thromboembolism, major bleeding, and death did not differ after 24 weeks of surveillance. The authors also evaluated quality of life, as perceived by their patients, and found that low molecular weight heparin use was associated with less impairment of physical activity and social functioning.

A second randomized clinical trial compared enoxaparin (1 mg/kg subcutaneously every 12 h) with inpatient continuous intravenous heparin [15]. Importantly, two-thirds of the eligible patients were excluded from participation. Reasons for exclusion included inability to receive outpatient therapy because of coexisting disease, patient refusal, symptomatic pulmonary embolism, prior thromboembolism, and geographic inaccessibility. Almost one-half of the patients assigned to enoxaparin were never admitted to the hospital, and a substantial fraction of patients were discharged after only a day or two in the hospital. Rates of recurrent venous thromboembolism (5.3% enoxaparin vs 6.7% heparin), major bleeding (2.0% enoxaparin vs 1.2% heparin), and mortality (4.5% enoxaparin vs 6.7% heparin) did not differ. However, two patients treated with enoxaparin suffered fatal bleeding complications, underscoring the importance of patient selection for outpatient management.

The results of these two studies suggest that physicians can treat many patients with acute proximal deep vein thrombosis safely with low molecular weight heparin given subcutaneously at home. Patient education, follow-up, and medications must be available and well organized in order for physicians and patients to realize the advantages of this advance. Patient selection is a very important consideration. Outpatient treatment for deep vein thrombosis is not appropriate for patients with symptomatic pulmonary embolism, increased risks for bleeding, or fatal pulmonary embolism; nor should it be used when the physician anticipates noncompliance. Although both clinical trials included patients with iliofemoral thrombosis, clinical decisions regarding outpatient treatment must take into account the severity of venous thrombosis and the availability of alternative therapies (e.g., thrombolysis) for patients with more severe disease.

Treatment of Acute Pulmonary Embolism

Although asymptomatic pulmonary embolism often accompanies symptomatic proximal deep vein thrombosis, physician-investigators excluded patients with symptomatic acute pulmonary embolism when they examined the safety and efficacy of low molecular weight heparins for the treatment of deep vein thrombosis. Thus it remained necessary to examine the effectiveness and safety of low molecular weight heparin preparations for the treatment of acute pulmonary embolism.

Two recently published studies have examined the effectiveness and safety of low molecular weight heparins for the treatment of acute pulmonary embolism [17, 19]. The first study, performed by a multinational consortium of investigators, compared reviparin with intravenous unfractionated heparin [17]. The study included patients with symptomatic venous thromboembolism ($n = 1021$). Unlike previous trials, patients with symptomatic pulmonary embolism ($n = 271$) were included. The overall rates of recurrent venous thromboembolism did not differ (5.3% reviparin vs 4.9% heparin); nor did major bleeding rates (3.1% reviparin vs 2.3% heparin) or mortality (7.1% reviparin vs 7.6% heparin). Among the 271 patients with symptomatic pulmonary embolism, symptomatic recurrence occurred with equal frequency in both groups (5.9%). However, this study fell short of proving equivalence between reviparin and unfractionated heparin for the treatment of acute pulmonary embolism because it did not have the power to detect clinically important differences in recurrence rates among patients with symptomatic acute pulmonary embolism.

A second unblinded randomized clinical trial compared tinzaparin (175 anti-Xa units/kg) with continuous intravenous heparin for a large number of patients ($n = 612$) with symptomatic acute pulmonary embolism [19]. Importantly, slightly more than half of the eligible patients were excluded, and the majority of patients received treatment with intravenous heparin before random assignment. A substantial number of patients were excluded by investigators because they had massive pulmonary embolism which may have required more aggressive treatment (e.g., thrombolysis or embolectomy). Similarly, many patients were excluded because they received more than 24 h of anticoagulant treatment before they could be entered into the trial. With these limitations, the investigators found no differences in the rates of recurrent venous thromboembolism (1.6% tinzaparin vs 1.9% heparin), major bleeding (2.0% tinzaparin vs 2.6% heparin), or death (3.9% tinzaparin vs 4.5% heparin).

These two trials suggest that low molecular weight heparins are as effective and safe as unfractionated heparin for the treatment of submassive acute pulmonary embolism.

Prophylaxis Against Venous Thromboembolism

General Surgery

General surgery patient populations are heterogeneous, and surgical techniques as well as postoperative care have evolved rapidly. Previous studies have suggested that 19% of patients who undergo general surgical procedures develop deep vein thrombi which can be confirmed by venography when prophylaxis against venous thromboembolism is withheld [20]. The incidence of deep vein thrombosis is greater in general surgical patients with malignant disease. Unfractionated heparin (5000 units subcutaneously every 8 or 12 h) effectively reduces the incidence of deep vein thrombosis following abdominal or pelvic surgical procedures [20].

A number of studies have compared low molecular weight heparins with unfractionated heparin for the prevention of venous thromboembolism following abdominal surgical procedures (Table 3). In the aggregate, these studies suggest that low molecular weight heparins are as effective as unfractionated

TABLE 3. Comparisons of low molecular weight heparins (LMWH) with unfractionated heparins (UH) for prevention of deep vein thrombi after abdominal surgery

First author, year [Ref.]	LMWH	Dose anti-Xaμ[a]	UH Dose Iμ	Deep vein thrombosis	
				LMWH	UH
Caen, 1988 [30]	Dalteparin	2500 qd	5000 b.i.d.	3.1	3.7
Bergqvist, 1988 [31]	Dalteparin	5000 qd	5000 b.i.d.	5.0*	9.2
Encke, 1988 [32]	Nadroparin	7500 qd	5000 t.i.d.	2.8*	4.5
Kakkar, 1997 [33]	Reviparin	1750 qd	5000 b.i.d.	4.7	4.3
Boneu, 1993 [34]	Reviparin	1750 qd	5000 b.i.d.	4.8	4.4
Nurmohamed, 1995 [35]	Enoxaparin	20 mg qd	5000 t.i.d.	8.1	6.3

[a] All doses administered subcutaneously 2 h preoperatively.
* P < 0.05.

heparin. Available evidence supports the use of larger doses for patients with malignancy who undergo abdominal surgery. Although low molecular weight heparins only require one injection each day, they are more expensive than unfractionated heparin and therefore it may be difficult to justify their routine use from an economic viewpoint.

Orthopedic Surgery

Deep vein thrombosis and pulmonary embolism are important causes of morbidity, mortality, and economic waste following total hip or total knee replacement. Without prophylaxis, deep vein thrombosis can be detected by contrast venography in 40% to 84% of patients who undergo these procedures [20]. However, symptomatic deep vein thrombosis and pulmonary embolism occur less frequently following these procedures.

The 1995 ACCP consensus conference [20] concluded that the choice among warfarin, low molecular weight heparin, and adjusted dose unfractionated heparin depended upon cost and convenience. Most orthopedic surgeons use warfarin.

Total Knee Replacement

Clinical trials have shown that low molecular weight heparins reduce rates of venographically detected deep vein thrombosis more effectively than warfarin (Table 4). One double-blind trial found that major bleeding was more frequent with low molecular weight heparin than with warfarin [21], underscoring the fine tradeoff between prevention of thrombosis and bleeding in this patient population.

Total Hip Replacement

Clinical trials have shown that low molecular weight heparins are as effective as warfarin in reducing rates of venographically detected deep vein thrombosis following total hip replacement (Table 5). Available evidence suggests that anti-

TABLE 4. Comparisons of low molecular weight heparins (LMWH) with warfarin (W) for prevention of deep vein thrombosis (DVT) after knee arthroplasty

First author, year [Ref.]	LMWH	Dose anti-Xaµ	DVT (%)		Major bleeding (%)	
			LMWH	W	LMWH	W
RD Heparin[a] group, 1994 [36]	Ardeparin	50 U/kg b.i.d.	26*	43	–	–
Hull, 1993 [21]	Tinzaparin	75 U/kg qd	45*	55	2.8	0.9
Leclerc, 1996 [37]	Enoxaparin	30 mg q 12 h	37*	52	–	–

[a] Denotes unilateral venography, all other investigators performed bilateral venography.
* Statistically significant reduction in the rate of DVT.

TABLE 5. Comparisons of low molecular weight heparins (LMWH) with warfarin (W) for prevention of deep vein thrombosis (DVT) after hip arthroplasty

First author, year [Ref.]	LMWH	Dose Anti Xaμ	DVT (%)		Major bleeding	
			LMWH	W	LMWH	W
RD Heparin[a] Group, 1994 [36]	Ardeparin	50 U/kg q 12 h	8	14	–	–
Hull, 1993 [21]	Tinzaparin	75 U/kg qd	21	23	1.5	2.8

[a] Denotes unilateral venography.

coagulant prophylaxis should be continued after hospital discharge [22, 23], although additional study of this issue appears warranted.

Multiple Trauma

Without prophylaxis, deep vein thrombi were detected by contrast venography in 58% of patients who had sustained major trauma [24]. Almost one-third of these patients had proximal deep vein thrombosis at the time of detection, and three patients suffered fatal pulmonary emboli before venography. Thus the incidence and severity of venous thromboembolism following major trauma provide a strong mandate for prophylaxis.

One randomized clinical trial [25] has shown that low molecular weight heparin (enoxaparin 30 mg subcutaneously every 12 h) prevents venous thrombosis more effectively than unfractionated heparin (5000 units subcutaneously every 12 h). This trial excluded patients with closed head injuries and bleeding on computed tomographic scan or uncontrolled bleeding from other sites of traumatic injury, underscoring the potential risks of anticoagulant prophylaxis after major trauma.

One small randomized clinical trial has suggested that low molecular weight heparin (tinzaparin, 3500 anti-Xa units subcutaneously every day) was more effective than unfractionated heparin (5000 units subcutaneously every 8 h) for patients with acute spinal cord injury [26].

Medical Conditions

As with general surgical procedures, medical patients represent a heterogeneous patient population, making generalizations difficult. Two randomized controlled trials suggest that low molecular weight heparin reduces the risk of venous thrombosis as effectively as unfractionated heparin for medical patients [27, 28].

Epidural or Spinal Hematomas

The United States Food and Drug Administration (FDA) issued a public health advisory to call attention to postmarketing reports of epidural or spinal hematomas when low molecular weight heparins are given concurrently with spinal/epidural anesthesia or spinal puncture. The incidence of this complication remains unknown. Many of the hematomas caused neurologic injury, including long-term or permanent paralysis. The FDA report notes that the majority of these complications occurred in elderly women undergoing orthopedic surgery, and that the risk was increased by the use of indwelling epidural catheters and by the concomitant use of drugs which affect hemostasis.

References

1. Fareed J, Walenga JM, Hoppensteadt D et al (1988) Comparative study on the in vitro and in vivo activities of seven low-molecular-weight heparins. Haemostasis 18:Suppl 3:3–15 [Erratum, Haemostasis 18:389a]
2. Young E, Prins M, Levine MN et al (1992) Heparin binding to plasma proteins, an important mechanism for heparin resistance. Thromb Haemost 67:639–643
3. Young E, Wells P, Holloway S (1994) Ex-vivo and in vitro evidence that low molecular weight heparins exhibit less binding to plasma proteins than unfractionated heparin. Thromb Haemost 71:300–3004
4. Barzu T, Molho P, Tobelem G et al (1985) Binding endocytosis of heparin by human endothelial cells in culture. Biochim Biophys Acta 845:196–203
5. Bjornsson TO, Wolfram KM, Kitchell BB (1982) Heparin kinetics determined by three assay methods. Clin Pharmacol Ther 31:104–113
6. Cadroy Y, Pourrat J, Baladre MF et al (1991) Delayed elimination of enoxaparin in patients with chronic renal insufficiency. Thromb Res 63:385–390
7. Carter CJ, Melton JG, Hirsch J et al (1982) The relationship between the hemorrhagic and antithrombotic properties of low molecular weight heparin in rabbits. Blood 59:1239–1245
8. Salzman EW, Rosenberg RD, Smith MH et al (1980) Effect of heparin and heparin fractions on platelet aggregation. J Clin Invest 65:64–73
9. Prandoni P, Lensing AWA, Buller HR et al (1992) Comparison of subcutaneous low-molecular-weight heparin with intravenous standard heparin in proximal deep-vein thrombosis. Lancet 339:441–445
10. Holm HA, Ly B, Handeland GF et al (1986) Subcutaneous heparin treatment of deep venous thrombosis: a comparison of unfractionated and low-molecular weight heparin. Haemostasis 16:30–37
11. Albada J, Niewenhuis HK, Sixma JJ (1989) Treatment of acute venous thromboembolism with low-molecular-weight heparin (Fragmin). Results of a double-blind randomized study. Circulation 80:935–940
12. Hull RD, Raskob GE, Pineo GF et al (1992) Subcutaneous low-molecular-weight heparin compared with continuous intravenous heparin in the treatment of proximal-vein thrombosis. N Engl J Med 326:975–982
13. Hull RD, Raskob GE, Rosenbloom D et al (1997) Treatment of proximal vein thrombosis with subcutaneous low-molecular-weight heparin vs. intravenous heparin. An economic perspective. Arch Intern Med 157:289–294
14. Lindmarker P, Holmstrom M, Granqvists S et al (1994) Comparison of once-daily subcutaneous Fragmin with continuous intravenous unfractionated heparin in the treatment of deep vein thrombosis. Thromb Haemost 72:186–190
15. Levine M, Gent M, Hirsh J et al (1996) A comparison of low-molecular-weight heparin administered primarily at home with unfractionated heparin administered in the hospital for proximal deep-vein thrombosis. N Engl J Med 334:677–681

16. Koopman MMW, Prandoni P, Piovella F et al (1996) Treatment of venous thrombosis with intravenous unfractionated heparin administered in the hospital as compared with subcutaneous low-molecular-weight heparin administered at home. N Engl J Med 334:682–687

17. The Columbus Investigators (1997) Low-molecular-weight heparin in the treatment of patients with venous thromboembolism. N Engl J Med 337:657–662

18. Lensing AWA, Prins MH, Davidson BL, Hirsh J (1995) Treatment of deep venous thrombosis with low-molecular-weight heparins: a meta-analysis. Arch Intern Med 155:601–607

19. Simonneau G, Sors H, Charbonnier B et al (1997) A comparison of low-molecular-weight heparin with unfractionated heparin for acute pulmonary embolism. N Engl J Med 337:663–669

20. Clagett GP, Anderson FA, Heit J et al (1995) Prevention of venous thromboembolism. Chest 108:Suppl:312S–334S

21. Hull R, Raskob G, Pineo G et al (1993) A comparison of subcutaneous low-molecular-weight heparin with warfarin sodium for prophylaxis against deep-vein thrombosis after hip or knee implantation. N Engl J Med 329:1370–1376

22. Planes A, Vochelle N, Darman JY et al (1996) Risk of deep venous thrombosis after hospital discharge in patients having undergone total hip replacement: double blind randomized comparison of enoxaparin versus placebo. Lancet 348:224–228

23. Bergqvist D, Benoni G, Bjorgell O et al (1996) Low-molecular-weight heparin (enoxaparin) as prophylaxis against venous thromboembolism after total hip replacement. N Engl J Med 335:696–700

24. Geerts WH, Code KI, Jay RM, Chen E, Szalai JP (1994) A prospective study of venous thromboembolism after major trauma. N Engl J Med 331:1601–1606

25. Geerts WH, Jay RN, Code KI et al (1996) A comparison of low-dose heparin with low-molecular-weight heparin as prophylaxis against venous thromboembolism after major trauma. N Engl J Med 335:701–707

26. Green D, Lee MY, Lim AC et al (1990) Prevention of thromboembolism after spinal cord injury using low-molecular-weight heparin. Ann Intern Med 113:571–574

27. Bergmann JF, Neuhart E (1996) A multicenter randomized double-blind study of enoxaparin compared with unfractionated heparin in the prevention of venous thromboembolic disease in elderly in-patients bedridden for an acute medical illness. Thromb Haemost 76:529–534

28. Harenberg J, Kallenbach B, Martin U et al (1990) Randomized controlled study of heparin and low molecular weight heparin for prevention of deep-vein thrombosis in medical patients. Thromb Res 59:639–650

29. Fiessinger JN, Lopez-Fernandez M, Gatterer E et al (1996) Once-daily subcutaneous dalteparin, a low-molecular-weight heparin, for the initial treatment of acute deep vein thrombosis. Thromb Haemost 76:195–199

30. Caen JP (1988) A randomized double-blind study between a low molecular weight heparin Kabi 2165 and standard heparin in the prevention of deep vein thrombosis in general surgery: a French multicenter trial. Thromb Haemost 59:216–220

31. Bergqvist D, Matzsch T, Burmark US et al (1988) Low molecular weight heparin given the evening before surgery compared with conventional low-dose heparin in prevention of thrombosis. Br J Surg 75:888–891

32. Encke A, Breddin K (1988) Comparison of a low-molecular-weight heparin and unfractionated heparin for the prevention of deep vein thrombosis in patients undergoing abdominal surgery. Br J Surg 75:1058–1063

33. Kakkar VV, Boeckl O, Boneu B et al (1997) Efficacy and safety of a low-molecular-weight heparin and standard unfractionated heparin for prophylaxis of postoperative venous thromboembolism: European multicenter trial. World J Surg 21:2–8
34. Boneu B (1993) An international multicenter study: clivarin in the prevention of venous thromboembolism in patients undergoing general surgery. Blood Coagul Fibrinolysis 4:Suppl 1:S21–S22
35. Nurmohamed MT, Verhaeghe R, Haas S et al (1995) A comparative trial of a low-molecular-weight heparin (enoxaparin) versus standard heparin for the prophylaxis of postoperative deep vein thrombosis. Am J Surg 169:567–571
36. RD Heparin Arthroplasty Group (1994) RD heparin compared with warfarin for prevention of venous thromboembolic disease following total hip or knee arthroplasty. J Bone Joint Surg Am 76:1174–1185
37. Leclerc JR, Geerts WH, Desjardins L et al (1996) Prevention of venous thromboembolism after knee arthroplasty: a randomized, double-blind trial comparing enoxaparin with warfarin. Ann Intern Med 124:619–626

Clinical Experience with Vena Caval Filters

Lazar J. Greenfield and Mary C. Proctor

Summary. The use of vena caval filters to prevent fatal pulmonary embolism (PE) has become the standard of care for patients who cannot be safely or effectively anticoagulated. This is due to several factors: improved devices, percutaneous methods of delivery, and long-term experience of safety and efficacy. Six vena caval filters are currently marketed with Food and Drug Administration approval: the Simon Nitinol, VenaTech, Bird's Nest, and three iterations of the Greenfield filter, Each of these devices has been reviewed based upon reports from published clinical studies. This type of summary is complicated by disparity in the study methodologies, numbers of patients, lengths of follow-up, and definition of adverse events. The need for established reporting standards is clear. A consensus document, which is in preparation, should be available in 1999 and should lead to greatly improved reports.

Keywords. Vena caval filter, Adverse events, Outcome, Pulmonary embolism

Vena caval interruption by means of a peripherally inserted filtration device dates to the 1960s with the use of the Mobin-Uddin caval umbrella. This device, which took its name from its umbrella shape, was effective in preventing emboli from reaching the pulmonary arteries but led to a 65% incidence of vena caval occlusion. It was withdrawn from the market following the introduction of a new device, the Greenfield filter (MediTech, Watertown, MA USA). This was a self-expanding cone-shaped device with six limbs held in place by curved hooks (Fig. 1). It was first described in 1973 [1] and has been in use since that time.

In the late 1980s, techniques for percutaneous venous access were developed which allowed the original Greenfield device to be placed without an operative procedure, thus reducing morbidity and cost. However, a large sheath was required for the 24 Fr carrier, adding the risk of insertion site thrombosis reported in from 5% to 41% [2, 3]. With a large potential patient population and improved

Department of Surgery, The University of Michigan, 2101 Taubman Center/Box 0346, Ann Arbor, MI 48109-0346, USA

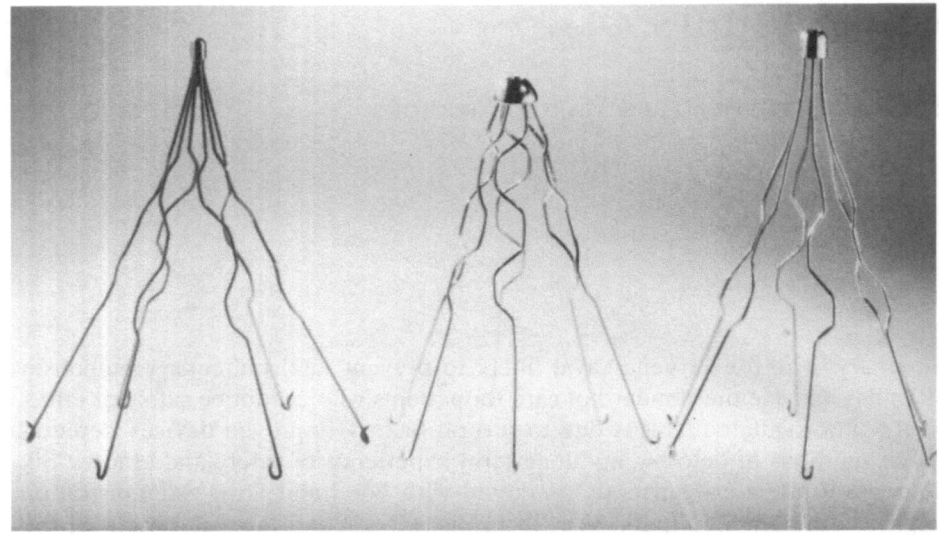

Fig. 1. The three Greenfield filters share a cone-shaped design which permits adequate flow in the vena cava despite the presence of large volumes of thrombus within the filter. The original stainless-steel model is shown in the *center*, the titanium model on the *left* and the percutaneous stainless-steel model on the *right*

technologies, three additional filters were evaluated and approved by the United States Food and Drug Administration (FDA). These devices include the Bird's Nest filter (BN) (Cook, Bloomington, IN USA) (Fig. 2), the VenaTech filter (VT) (Braun, Evanston, IL USA) (Fig. 3), and the Simon Nitinol filter (SN) (Nitinol Medical, Woburn, MA) (Fig. 4). Two modified versions of the Greenfield filter for percutaneous placement, one of titanium (TGF) and one of stainless steel (PSGF), also received FDA approval in 1990 and 1996, respectively (see Fig. 1).

As new devices began to gain clinical acceptance, authors began to redefine the characteristics of an ideal filter. Grassi and Goldhaber [4] identified six desirable characteristics: biocompatibility, filtering efficiency, flow maintenance, rapid percutaneous insertion, secure fixation, and retrievability. Yune reduced this list of "ideal" qualities to five: low incidence of caval thrombosis, division of the cava into "multiple small lumens" by a simple device, placement ease without major surgery, secure placement in the desired position and orientation, and retrievability. Ten years later, developers are still striving to accomplish these objectives.

The volume of literature devoted to vena caval filters has significantly increased over time, reflecting the growing acceptance of this intervention. Three topics account for the bulk of the increase: case reports of adverse events, controversial indications for placement, and new investigational devices. Several authors have also published review articles characterizing existing devices. These have emphasized early outcomes of patients with various devices [5–7]. Some are a synthesis of oral and written reports [8] or review articles [9–11], while others

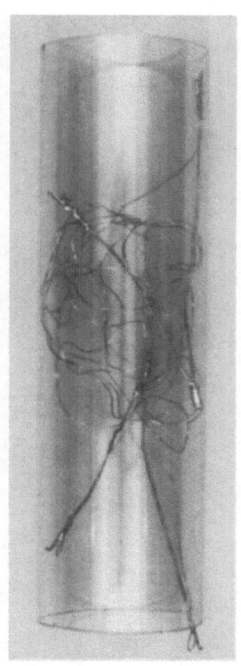

FIG. 2. The Bird's Nest filter is free-formed within a 6–7 cm segment of the vena cava. It may be used in cavas greater than 28 mm

are descriptive of filter placement [12, 13]. These reports are useful for physicians wishing to gain general knowledge regarding various filters but do not provide comprehensive information. To understand both the strengths and limitations of the devices, it is necessary to examine publications which report the results of prospective clinical evaluation, preferably from the FDA approval studies.

The LGM or VenaTech filter is a cone-shaped device stamped from Phylox which is a combination of cobalt, chromium, iron, nickel, and traces of other metals. In addition to the cone, six vertical struts are welded to the legs and a sharp barb is added to the tip. The struts are intended to center the filter within the vena cava and to attach it to the caval wall (Fig. 3).

The initial clinical studies were performed in France and reported by Ricco et al. [14] (Table 1). In this well-designed study, 100 patients with an objective diagnosis of pulmonary embolism (85%) or proximal deep vein thrombosis (DVT) (15%) received a VenaTech filter. Physical examination and vena cavography were obtained on day 8 and then 3, 6, and 12 months following placement. When possible, all patients received intravenous heparin following filter placement and were given oral anticoagulants for 3 months. These same investigators performed follow-up 6 years later and found a similar rate of recurrent PE, but a significant increase in caval occlusion (30%) accompanied by a 59% incidence of lower extremity edema.

Reports from three studies in the United States have also been published. Taylor et al. [15] reviewed 81 patients with follow-up ranging from 5 to 568 days.

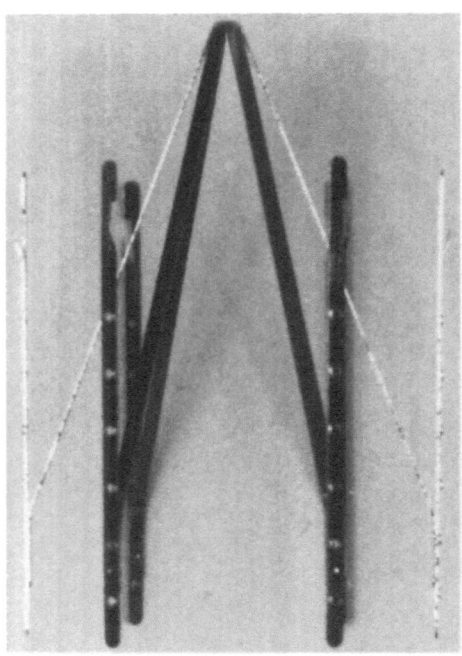

FIG. 3. The VenaTech filter adds six side struts to the cone to improve centering within the vena cava

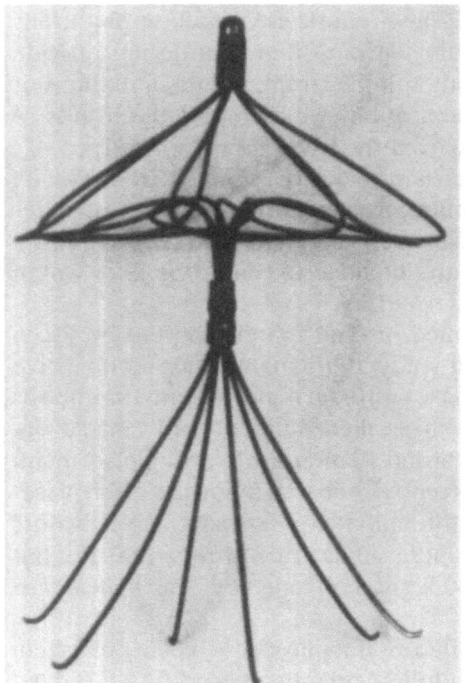

FIG. 4. The Simon Nitinol filter is the smallest of the approved devices. The petal-shaped dome adds a second level of protection

TABLE 1. Summary of published reports on the use of vena caval filters

	VT [14]	VT [42]	VT [15]	BN [19]	SN[b]	SGF [32]	TGF [33]	TGF [34]	PSGF [37]
Duration	1 year	6 years	4 months	5 years	6 months	20 years	30 days	>12 months	30 days
No. entered	100	146	101	568	273	642	186	173	75
No. of filters placed	98	142	97	568	273	667	181	173	75
Deaths	8	53	18	NR	84	280	35	21	8
No. with follow-up	90	137		440	162	246	123	92	60
PE	2%	3.6%	0%	2.9%	3%	4%	3%	3.5%	0
IVC Occlusion	7%	30%	8%	2.9%	18%	4%	NR	1%	5%
Asymmetry	NR[c]	NR	NR	NR	NR	NR	5.4%	10%	5%
Incomplete opening	8%	NR	6%	NR	NR	NR	2%	NR	1.3%
Tilt	11%	0.8%	2%	NR	25%[a]	5%	NR	NR	NR
Malposition	16%	NR	3%	NR	NR	2%	1%	2.8%	0
Migration	13%	16%	12%	1%	0.7%	5%	11%	7.6%	0
Lower extremity edema	29%	59%	NR	NR	NR	5%	10%	22%	0

Number in brackets indicates ref. no. VT, VenaTech; BN, Bird's Nest; SN, Simon Nitinol; SGF, stainless-steel Greenfield; TGF, titancium Greenfield; PSGF, percutaneons stainless-steel Greenfield; PE, pulmonary embolism; IVC, inferion vena cava; NR, not reported.

[a] Dome tilted.

[b] Robert Brown (President, Nitinol Technologies), personal communication.

The position of the filter remained stable in two-thirds of patients but one filter was fractured 10 months following placement. Data regarding recurrent PE in 53 patients were assessed by chart review and interview. Two patients had objective confirmation of recurrent PE (2/53) for an incidence of 3.7%. Vena caval patency was documented in 30/33 patients or 90%. One of the characteristics of all three occluded filters was a noticeable narrowing at the base, resulting in a collapsed appearance. The authors also indicated that they were not able to image thrombus within the filter using duplex ultrasound. One of the major shortcomings of this study was the lack of a standardized protocol. The timing and type of diagnostic study varied among the participating centers, making the analysis very difficult to interpret.

A second study of the VenaTech filter was conducted concurrently by Murphy et al. [16]. Filters were successfully placed in 97 patients with a 6% incidence of incomplete opening. Insertion site venous patency was 67%, and 37% of the filters contained thrombus which extended proximally beyond the filter in 20%. These findings were noted between 1 day and 40 weeks following placement among the 35 patients studied (Table 1). Although the authors indicate that there was no recurrent PE, two patients had positive V/Q scans, one patient who died during the procedure may have had PE per their report, and a final death among those with only clinical evaluation may have been due to PE. There were five cases of decreased filter base diameter greater than 7 mm, four of whom had thrombus in the filter.

Millward et al. [17] studied 63 VenaTech filter patients and found similar success with placement but slightly higher rates of recurrent PE (6%), one of which was fatal. Their study differed from that of Murphy in the high incidence of caval occlusion (28%) of which 12 were symptomatic. There were also two reports of proximal propagation of thrombus. Only four migrations were seen but they ranged from 23–47 mm, which is greater than in other reports.

The Bird's Nest filter is the only one of the marketed devices that does not use the cone design and that can be placed in cavas greater than 28 mm in diameter (Fig. 2). It was developed in response to perceived problems encountered with earlier devices. It is constructed of four stainless-steel wires attached to two sets of hooks that secure it to the vena cava. Two hooks are placed followed by preformed wires which are arranged in the vena cava by the operator. The final two hooks are deployed in juxtaposition to the others to gain maximum compression of the wires and to minimize the open spaces to ensure a tight filtration grid [18]. Outcomes from the initial series of patients were disturbing as there were six cases in which the filter migrated to the right heart or the pulmonary artery. The final case resulted in death. This design problem was addressed by changing to an inflexible strut of 0.46 mm which necessitated an increase in size of the insertion system from 8 to 12 Fr [19].

Roehm et al. reported data for 440 Bird's Nest filter patients with at least 6 months of follow-up. The clinical outcomes were obtained by telephone conversations with the patient, family, or physician, or by a questionnaire. Information regarding clinical course, pulmonary embolism, vena caval occlusion, and cause of death was obtained. The criteria for complications consisted of the absence of new leg swelling, hemoptysis, and unexplained chest pain. Objective data were rare (Table 1). Of 27 cavograms, six were occluded for an incidence of 22%. Ultrasound results showed 1 of 10 patients with occlusion, and one of three pulmonary angiograms was positive for new PE. The interview follow-up of 440 patients ranging from 6 months to 5 years found 12 recurrent PE (2.7%) and 13 caval occlusions (2.9%) [18]. Determining event rates from a study that only had objective follow-up in 10% of the patients is not valid. Diagnostic studies were obtained only in symptomatic cases, creating biased estimates of the variables. There are also problems with underestimation of events among those not studied.

The incidence of insertion site thrombosis was not addressed in the study by Roehm and coworkers, but Hicks et al. examined 48 patients who had BN filters placed 1 to 11 days earlier, and 10 patients had either occlusive or nonocclusive thrombus for an incidence of 21%. There was no extension of thrombus among the nine with nonocclusive thrombus [20]. The BN filter requires more operator control than the other devices and therefore an awareness of the potential problems.

Vesely et al. placed 165 BN filters over a period of 16 months and reported five potential problems. If the infrarenal IVC is short, there may be insufficient space for forming the wire mesh, making site selection difficult. When the angle of the iliac vein is acute, the sheath may kink after the introducer is removed. This occurred in 5% of cases. Attempts to force the filter through a kinked sheath can result in damage to the vein. In 8% of cases, cephalad prolapse of the wires was observed. This was more common in patients with short infrarenal segments. The effect of wire prolapse on filtering efficiency is unknown. Prior to redesign of the delivery system, problems were also encountered with release of the filter. A new delivery system is intended to correct this liability. Another problem was experienced as the guide wire pusher was released and withdrawn which should also be addressed by the new delivery system [21]. Other than the initial questionnaire data reported by Roehm et al., there have been few outcome studies in the literature for patients with this filter. Two small series, one from Australia [22] and one from Toronto [23], report objective follow-up in a total of 51 patients. No recurrent PE or caval occlusions were detected. Five patients had thrombus in the filter which was not occlusive. Twelve patients underwent computed tomography (CT) examination and in all cases, the inferior vena cava (IVC) was penetrated by the struts. Penetrations ranged from 5 to 19mm and involved the psoas muscle, aorta, common iliac artery, duodenum, pancreas, and a vertebral body, all of which were asymptomatic. The studies of this filter are limited by one of two factors: lack of objective follow-up [19] or inadequate sample size [23, 24]. It is of interest that the reported complications were the same as those that initially led to dissatisfaction with the existing devices.

The Simon Nitinol filter has the advantage of having the smallest delivery size (9 Fr) of all the filters which allows for percutaneous placement via the antecubital vein [25]. The smaller system is achieved through the use of an innovative metal, Nitinol, an alloy of nickel and titanium (Fig. 4). This material has "thermal memory," allowing it to be stored in the delivery system as straight wire but assuming its preformed cone-petal shape when placed in the vena cava [26]. The filter has two components: a lower six-legged cone similar to the other devices and a proximal seven petal-shaped dome. The two structures work together for increased thrombus trapping efficiency.

The SN filter was evaluated in a 26-center clinical study involving 273 patients. Patients were studied 3 and 6 months following placement by means of plain films: magnetic resonance imaging (MRI), ultrasound, and V/Q scans were used in some cases. To our knowledge, the final report of this study remains unpublished. A written personal communication from Robert Brown, President of Nitinol Medical Technologies from July of 1991, forms the basis of this report (Table 1). The incidence of recurrent PE was 4% and occlusion of the IVC was found in 18%. It is not possible to determine how many patients underwent objective testing. A publication by Kim et al. [27] involving some of the investigators in the clinical trial performed during the same time period suggests the number was only 18. We are unaware of any clinical study in a large group of patients with long-term outcome data. A group of 24 consecutive patients with SN filters were enrolled at two centers were underwent physical examination, ten went on to MRI to evaluate uni- or bilateral lower extremity swelling. Vena caval occlusion was identified in five of the ten cases, all of whom had a malignancy [26]. A report from the University of Arkansas provided outcomes for a group of 16 patients with a mean follow-up of 14 months. There were no recurrent PE but there were five caval penetrations, four caval thromboses, one migration, and two filter leg fractures [28].

The Greenfield vena caval filter has the longest history of follow-up among the currently available devices. The original stainless-steel filter was described by Greenfield et al. [29] in 1973. Outcome data have been reported at frequent intervals [30, 31] with the most recent report in 1995 [32] (Table 1). This study had a mean follow-up time of 53 months. The incidence of recurrent PE and caval occlusion was 4% and there was no deterioration of results over time when compared to the 5- and 12-year reports.

To decrease morbidity from insertion site thrombosis and facilitate percutaneous placement, a reduced profile Greenfield filter was developed. It was manufactured from titanium, a material with a high elastic characteristic which allows it to regain its original size and shape when released from the carrier. The titanium Greenfield filter (TGF) was initially tested in a group of 50 patients and found to function well as a filter but to have inadequate fixation. The hooks underwent modification, and a multicenter study of the new design was conducted. This filter is slightly longer (4.7 cm) and has a wider resting base diameter (3.8 cm vs 3.0 cm) than the standard filter. The rate of recurrent PE was only 3% and fixation was greatly improved with a migration rate of 11% [33] (Table 1). This report led to FDA approval in 1990.

To determine whether the performance of the TGF was durable over a longer period of time, a second study was conducted in 173 patients with at least 12 months of follow-up in 113 patients, 85 of whom had participated in the previously cited study (Table 1). The 3.5% rate of recurrent PE and the high caval patency rate of 99% after 12 months suggested that the TGF is at least comparable to if not more effective than the original filter [34]. (Table 1). One concern with this design involved the occasional uneven spacing of the limbs of the filter at placement [35], suggesting a possible decrease in clot-trapping efficiency. An in vitro study was conducted to determine whether there was an association between leg spacing and clot trapping. The results failed to find a statistically significant association between these variables. Moreover, caval size was demonstrated to be the major factor associated with trapping efficacy [36]. This in vitro conclusion has been supported by clinical results [34].

The titanium Greenfield filter was designed for placement through a sheath, but its design precluded the stabilizing effect of a guidewire. Since the guidewire provides valuable assistance for introduction and centering of the filter carrier, a percutaneous stainless-steel filter was developed to allow passage through tortuous vessels, alignment of the carrier within the IVC, and improved centering within the vena cava. This device is manufactured from the same material as the original SGF but the leg extends from the apex at a $0°$ angle vs $17°$ with the standard filter. This allows it to be compressed into a 12 Fr delivery system. It also differs from the SGF and TGF in that two of the hooks are angled downward to improve fixation. The filter is the longest of the Greenfield designs (4.9 cm) with a base of 3.2 cm. In the initial FDA study, the major outcome criteria, as determined from AP and lateral plain films, were fixation and caval penetration. This study showed no migration greater than 20 mm and only three cases in which the filter base increased by more than 5 mm. Two cases had penetration ruled out by CT and the third was not definitive, for a penetration rate of 1.7%. Three patients at one center presented with caval occlusion by ultrasound, but no further studies were performed as all were end-stage cancer patients. No other patients were examined for patency during the study and no clinical pulmonary embolism occurred [37] (Table 1). This publication also contains data on a small group of patients with a longer period of follow-up. Among these nine patients, there was no PE but one new DVT occurred. All insertion sites were patent. There was no migration but one probable penetration. All patients had duplex ultrasound studies of the IVC. Eight of the nine were able to be interpreted and all were patent [37].

The choice of a filter should be made on the basis of long-term performance, as these are permanently implanted devices which can result in significant morbidity and mortality if they fail. Despite the compelling need for cost control, this is a decision that should be made by a physician rather than a financial administrator.

The major criteria for selection of a particular vena caval filter must include its efficacy and safety. The fundamental purpose of a filter is to prevent significant pulmonary embolism. While it is not necessary to trap all tiny emboli, the device must be able to prevent fatal PE. For this criterion, all of the devices appear to perform in a similar fashion. With over 20 years of objective follow-up with the

Greenfield filter, we have seen a consistent PE rate of 2%–4% [32, 34]. Clinical or survey follow-up of the other devices has been similar [15, 22, 38].

The second criterion is patency of the vena cava. The challenge in designing a filter is to balance a high rate of clot capture with a high rate of caval patency. Devices can be designed with more metal structure to capture all emboli, but at the price of reduced caval patency. Alternatively, flow can be maintained but with risk of loss of smaller emboli. Reduction in flow can develop in two ways: obstruction due to the presence of trapped thrombus in which case the filter has performed well, or actual reduction in caval diameter related to stricture from endothelial or myointimal hyperplasia. This ingrowth may be a reaction to the amount of metal in contact with the vessel wall and the pressure on it, or there may be contraction of the wall in response to thrombus contracture. In either case, the patient may develop increased distal venous pressure and chronic venous insufficiency.

Three of the four vena caval filters share a conical design and are intended for use in a cava of 28 mm diameter or less. Only the Bird's Nest filter is free-form and can be used in abnormally large cavas. When the cava measures in excess of 35 mm after correcting for magnification error, the options include use of the Bird's Nest filter or standard filters in both iliac veins.

In some patients it may be difficult to find an appropriate insertion site due to the presence of thrombus in the femoral veins and central lines in the jugular veins. In this case, the Simon Nitinol filter may be able to be inserted through an antecubital vein as it only requires a 9 Fr insertion system [25]. Similarly, the presence of thrombus may limit the length of cava in which a filter may be deployed. In these cases, the original stainless-steel Greenfield filter may be the device of choice as it is the shortest. Finally, when the filter is to be placed in the suprarenal vena cava, any of the Greenfield filters should be selected as they are the only devices with a long history of patency in this location [31, 39, 40].

There has been considerable interest in a temporary filter although none is available for marketing. The major perceived advantage is that the patient would not be left with a permanently implanted device. Prototypes have been developed and used in Europe, but several issues remain to be addressed. The period during which patients remain at risk of PE remains unknown, but has been suggested to be as long as 6 weeks following elective orthopedic procedures and longer than that in patients with spinal cord injuries. The limit of opportunity for device removal appears to be 3 to 4 weeks at maximum when fixation to the wall of the cava makes removal difficult and potentially damaging. If the device captures a thrombus, it is unclear as to how it can be safely removed without risk of embolism and whether a permanent device is required. Devices which require an external tether also leave the patient at risk for sepsis. There is certainly no economic advantage in using a temporary filter, as the procedural cost of placing the device is comparable to placement of a permanent filter and there is an additional procedural cost for removal. Finally, if there were adverse events related to the long-term presence of a vena caval filter, the case for a temporary device would be strengthened, but we have followed patients with the original 24 Fr

Greenfield filter since 1972 [32] and have found that the long-term outcomes did not differ from the earlier reports [30, 31, 41]. These data make the utility of a temporary filter negligible.

The choice of a vena caval filter becomes simple if the literature is reviewed. Long-term, objective outcome studies should be the ultimate guide. While small series with limited data are available for all of the caval filters, larger series with objective follow-up have been published only for the VenaTech [17, 42] and Greenfield filters [34, 43]. A careful reading of these studies is the responsibility of every physician who inserts vena caval filters.

References

1. Elkins R, McCurdy J, Brown P, Greenfield LJ (1973) Clinical results with an extracaval prosthesis and description of a new intracaval filter. J Oklahoma State Med Assoc 53–59
2. Tobin KD, Pais O, Austin CB (1989) Femoral vein thrombosis following percutaneous placement of the Greenfield filter. Invest Radiol 24:442–445
3. Pais O, Mirvis S, De Orchis D (1987) Percutaneous insertion of the Kimray-Greenfield filter: technical considerations and problems. Radiology 165:377–381
4. Grassi CJ, Goldhaber SZ (1989) Interruption of the inferior vena cava for prevention of pulmonary embolism: transvenous filter devices. Herz 14(3):182–191
5. Aswad MA, Sandager GP, Pais SO et al (1996) Early duplex scan evaluation of four vena caval interruption devices. J Vasc Surg 24(5):809–818
6. Redhead DN, Adam R, Allan P, Ruckley CV (1989) Radiological evaluation of caval patency and filter migration in patients with caval interruption/filtration. J Intervent Radiol 4:42–45
7. Mohan CR, Hoballah JJ, Sharp WJ, Kresowik T, Lu CT, Corson JD (1995) Comparative efficacy and complications of vena caval filters. J Vasc Surg 21(2):235–246
8. Dorfman GS (1990) Percutaneous inferior vena caval filters. Radiology 174(2):987–992
9. Becker D, Philbrick J, Selby JB (1992) Inferior vena cava filters: indications, safety, effectiveness. Arch Intern Med 152:1985–1994
10. Grassi CJ (1991) Inferior vena caval filters: analysis of five currently available devices. AJR 156:813–821
11. Redhead DN (1993) Inferior vena caval filters. J Intervent Radiol 8:121–126
12. Grassi CJ (1994) Inferior vena caval filters: percutaneous use and types. In: Taversas JM, Ferrucci JT (eds) Radiology. Diagnosis—imaging—intervention. Lippincott, Philadelphia, pp 1–10
13. Ballew KA, Philbrick JT, Becker DM (1995) Vena cava filter devices. Clin Chest Med 16(2):295–305
14. Ricco JB, Crochet DP Sebilotte P et al (1988) Percutaneous transvenous caval interruption with xLGMx filter. Ann Vasc Surg 2:242–247
15. Taylor FC, Awh MH, Kahn CE, Lu CT (1991) Vena Tech vena cava filter: experience and early follow-up. JVIR 2:435–440
16. Murphy TP, Dorfman GS, Yedlicka JW et al (1991) LGM vena cava filter: objective evaluation of early results. JVIR 2:107–115
17. Millward S, Peterson R, Moher D et al (1994) LGM (Vena Tech) vena caval filter: experience at a single institution. JVIR 5:351–356

18. Roehm J, Gianturco C, Barth M (1985) Percutaneous interruption of the inferior vena cava: The Bird's Nest filter. In: Bergan J, Yao J (eds) Surgery of the Veins. Grune and Stratton, Orlando, 481–495
19. Roehm J, Johnsrude I, Barth M, Gianturco C (1988) The Birdxs Nest inferior vena cava filter: progress report. Radiology 168(3):745–749
20. Hicks M, Middleton W, Picus D, Darcy M, Kleinhoffer M (1990) Prevalence of local venous thrombosis after transfemoral placement of a bird's nest vena caval filter. JVIR 1:63–68
21. Vesely T, Darcy M, Picus D, Hicks M (1992) Technical problems associated with placement of the Bird's Nest inferior vena cava filter. AJR 158(4):875–880
22. Lord R, Benn I (1994) Early and late results after Bird's Nest filter placement in the inferior vena cava: clinical and duplex ultrasound follow up. Aust NZ J Surg 64(2):106–114
23. Starok MS, Common AA (1996) Follow-up after insertion of Bird's Nest inferior vena caval filters. Can Assoc Radiol J 47:189–194
24. Alpert JS, Smith RB, Ockene I, Askenazik J, Dexter K, Dalen JE (1975) Treatment of massive pulmonary embolism: the role of pulmonary embolectomy. Am Heart J 89:413–418
25. Kim D, Schlam B, Porter DH, Simon M (1991) Insertion of the Simon Nitinol caval filter: value of the antecubital vein approach. AJR 157:521–522
26. Grassi CJ, Matsumoto A, Teitelbaum G (1992) Vena caval occlusion after Simon Nitinol filter placement: identification with MR imaging in patients with malignancy. JVIR 3:535–539
27. Kim D, Edelman R, Margolin C et al (1992) The Simon Nitinol filter: evaluation by MR and ultrasound. Angiology 43(7):541–548
28. McCowan T, Ferris E, Carver DK, Molpus WM (1992) Complications of the nitinol vena caval filter. JVIR 3:401–408
29. Greenfield LJ, McCurdy J, Brown P, Elkins R (1973) A new intracaval filter permitting continued flow and resolution of emboli. Surgery 73:599–606
30. Greenfield LJ, Peyton R, Crute S, Barnes RW (1981) Greenfield vena caval filter experience: Late results in 156 patients. Arch Surg 116:1451–1455
31. Greenfield LJ, Michna B (1988) Twelve-year clinical experience with the Greenfield vena caval filter. Surgery 104(4):706–712
32. Greenfield LJ, Proctor MC (1995) Twenty-year clinical experience with the Greenfield filter. Cardiovasc Surg 3(2):199–205
33. Greenfield LJ, Cho KJ, Proctor MC et al (1991) Results of a multicenter study of the modified hook titanium Greenfield filter. J Vasc Surg 14:253–257
34. Greenfield LJ, Proctor MC, Cho KJ et al (1994) Extended evaluation of the titanium Greenfield vena caval filter. J Vasc Surg 20:458–465
35. Vesely T (1994) Technical problems and complications associated with inferior vena cava filters. Semin Intervent Radiol 11(2):121–133
36. Greenfield LJ (1994) Assessment of asymmetric opening of the Titanium Greenfield Filter. JVIR 5(3):528–529
37. Cho KJ, Greenfield LJ, Proctor MC et al (1997) Evaluation of a new percutaneous stainlesssteel Greenfield filter. JVIR 8:181–187
38. Hawkins SP, Al-Kutoubi A (1992) The Simon nitinol inferior vena cava filter: preliminary experience in the UK. Clin Radiol 46:378–380
39. Stewart J, Peyton W, Crute S, Greenfield LJ (1982) Clinical results of suprarenal placement of the Greenfield vena cava filter. Surg 92(1):1–4

40. Greenfield LJ, Cho KJ, Proctor MC, Sobel M, Shah S, Wingo J (1992) Late results of suprarenal Greenfield vena cava filter placement. Arch Surg 127:969–973
41. Greenfield LJ, Proctor MC, James EA, Abrams GD, Moursi MM (1994) Staging of fixation and retrievability of Greenfield filters. J Vasc Surg 20(5):744–750
42. Crochet DP, Stora O, Ferry D et al (1993) Vena Tech-LGM filter: long-term results of a prospective study. Radiology 188:857–860
43. Kniemeyer HW, Sandmann W (1990) Extended indications for placement of an inferior vena cava filter. J Vasc Surg 12(1):105–107

Subject Index